Into the House of Old

MCGILL-QUEEN'S ASSOCIATED MEDICAL SERVICES
(HANNAH INSTITUTE) Studies in the History of Medicine,
Health, and Society Series Editors: S.O. Freedman and J.T.H. Connor

Volumes in this series have financial support from Associated Medical Services, Inc., through the Hannah Institute for the History of Medicine program.

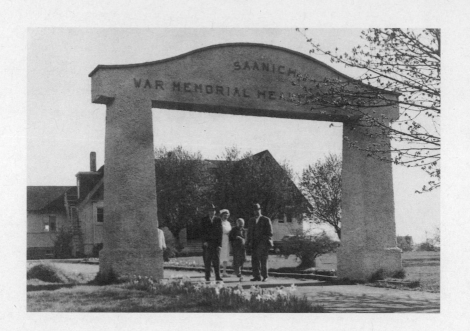

Into the House of Old

A History of Residential Care in British Columbia

MEGAN J. DAVIES

McGill-Queen's University Press
Montreal · Kingston · London · Ithaca

© McGill-Queen's University Press 2003
ISBN 0-7735-2502-5 (cloth)
ISBN 0-7735-2645-5 (pbk)

Legal deposit second quarter 2003
Bibliothèque nationale du Québec

Printed in Canada on acid-free paper that is 100%
ancient forest free (100% post-consumer recycled),
processed chlorine free.

This book has been published with the help of a grant
from the Humanities and Social Sciences Federation
of Canada, using funds provided by the Social Sciences
and Humanities Research Council of Canada.

McGill-Queen's University Press acknowledges the
support of the Canada Council for the Arts for our
publishing program. We also acknowledge the financial
support of the Government of Canada through the Book
Publishing Industry Development Program (BPIDP) for
our publishing activities.

National Library of Canada Cataloguing in Publication

Davies, Megan Jean, 1959–
    Into the house of old: a history of residential care
    in British Columbia/Megan J. Davies.

    (McGill-Queen's/Associated Medical Services (Hannah
    Institute) studies in the history of medicine, health,
    and society; no. 14)
    Includes bibliographical references and index.
    ISBN 0-7735-2502-5 (bnd); ISBN 0-7735-2645-5 (pbk)
    1. Old age homes – British Columbia – History. 1. Title.
    II. Series.
    RA998.C3D39 2003   362.1'6'09711   C2002-905041-3

Typeset in Sabon 10/12
by Caractéra inc., Quebec City

Contents

Tables and Figures

Illustrations

Acknowledgments

This book is based on my Ph.D. thesis, revised over many years with little blood but much sweat, a few tears, and considerable juggling of babysitting schedules. I thank the Hannah Institute for the History of Medicine for their continued support: this wouldn't be a book had I not received funding. I thank the Centre for the History of Medicine (Wellcome Unit), University of Glasgow, for providing me with a professional home. I was fortunate to have Andrée Lévesque as my supervisor at McGill University and to have extremely useful comments about the dissertation from Brian Young and Colin Howell. The kindness of fate delivered to me two incredibly supportive mentors: Jean Barman of the University of British Columbia and Marguerite Dupree of the University of Glasgow never stopped encouraging me toward the goal of turning thesis into book. It gives me great pleasure to thank them in print. I would also like to thank the two scholars who reviewed my work for their fine suggestions, and Lesley Barry for her excellent and engaged reworking of the manuscript. Staff at the following archives and institutions gave assistance: British Columbia Archives, British Columbia Legislative Library, Diocese of British Columbia Archives, Gorge Road Hospital, National Archives of Canada, National Library of Canada, Rose Manor, Oak Bay Municipal Clerk's Office, Saanich Municipal Archives, Simmons College Archives, Sisters of Saint Ann Archives, University of Toronto Archives, Victoria City Archives, and Vancouver City Archives. Sheila Norton, then at B.C.'s provincial archive, gave key input in the first stages of my research. Rolf Knight provided valuable feedback about single elderly men in B.C. and generously shared one of his personal photographs. David Havard kindly allowed for the use of his childhood snapshots: his memoirs of growing up in Victoria's Old Men's Home are an invaluable link with a past era. Dorthy Nora Mason (née Bentley), Barbara L.F. Wassersleben (née Bentley), and Peggy Lou Bentley-Stoffels (née Bentley) – descendants of Percy Bentley – heard my wish to use his beautiful portrait of "The Prospecter" and made it so. Richard Mackie helped out with sources in the early stages. Ariel Rogers graciously gave me permission me to quote from one of Stan Rogers' songs – thanks from a fan. These wonderful women took loving care of my children, freeing me to write without guilt: Denise Gareau, Aimie and Helen Brown, Sheila Van Leishout, Jennifer McTaggert, Ruth Lancaster, Corinna Pugh, and Christina Lynch.

Some debts go a long way back. My mother, Brenda Davies, gave me the love I needed right from the beginning. The incredible courage with which she has faced each day of the past decade moves me to tears – and then inspires me to do the best I can in my life. Not many teenagers get to attend a Great Battles in History Lecture Series with their dad, but I did. I want to thank John Davies for loving history and for loving me. My grandfather, George Barret Davies, spoilt me rotten and taught me that history is about real people. Two truly great aunts – Anna Martin and Rachel Coates – opened my mind to the experience of being female and elderly. I would like to acknowledge the support that I have received for this project from other important elders in my life: Peggy Baker, Yvonne Coggins, Gerry Grant, and Margaret Thorburn.

During the time I was working on this book my cast of beloved female friends have fed me, laughed with me, picked up the pieces when I have fallen apart, cared for my kids, upgraded my wardrobe, listened to me talk about my work, picked me up at the airport, and driven me to the ferry. In order of appearance: Michele Billung-Meyer, Susan Williams, Tracy Lynch, Karen Truscott, Margot Harrison, Olive Mann, Moira Coady, Sally Gose, Rosebud Morgan, Barb Grantham, Rose Stanton, Tamara Myers, Maureen Malowany, Nicole Matiation, Jenny Head, Lucy Hunter, Carey Morning, Ruth Sandwell, Lucila Machado, Mimo Caenepeel, Anna Shepherd, and Anne Fyfe. To Olive – a loving thank you for sharing your home while I did my initial research. And to Evan Mann – thanks for the chance for a little post-archival wrestling. Carey, sister-in-exile, gave me not just a room but a big beautiful sunlit flat of my own – a birthing place for this book. Bless you dear friend.

But it is the folks whom I breakfast with each morning that deserve the biggest thanks. Colin Coates has done so much on the practical level but, most important, I am daily inspired by his integrity as an historian, father, and life-partner. His faith in my creativity, even if it isn't bringing in a paycheque, has been critical. Mothering our children, Mab Yvonne and Bryn Garnet Richard, jarred me loose from an academic mindset and allowed me to re-discover the power of pulling people out of the past and putting their lives on the printed page. Bryn, Mab, and Colin – your love lets me dance as if no one is watching. This book is dedicated to you with my whole heart.

Into the House of Old

Introduction:
The House of Old

Some years ago, walking through an unfamiliar section of Victoria, British Columbia, I took an illicit shortcut and found myself at the entrance to the nursing home where my grandmother spent the final months of her life. In an instant I was twelve years old again, submerged in my grandfather's grief, horrified by the flimsy curtains meant to offer patients a measure of privacy, and sickened by the smell of stale urine. I had visited the place only once, yet the experience was indelibly etched on my emotional map.

I am not alone in this response to institutions for the elderly. On learning that I was writing about nursing homes, many people have shared sad and sometimes tragic tales about placing aged kin in residential accommodation. In western culture the old age home is *always* a place of deep loss, best avoided. *"Get me out of here,"* says the father to his daughter in Margaret Atwood's searing poem "King Lear in Respite Care."[1] Hagar Shipley, the elderly protagonist of Margaret Laurence's *The Stone Angel*, runs away rather than enter a nursing home.[2] The institution is impersonal and sterile, ultimately only a place of death. A widower in folk singer Stan Rogers' song "First Christmas" seeks out the common room in his new residence, where "they've got the biggest tree, and it's huge and cold and lifeless, not like it ought to be."[3] Most academic studies of the old age home are similarly negative. My generation, raised in the 1960s and 1970s, baulks at the regimentation and compulsion that are features of the institutional experience, turning easily to Michel Foucault's and Erving Goffman's notions of social control and the total institution.

Yet I believe that our rejection of residential care for the elderly has deeper cultural roots. Those interested in today's old age home have to look further back in history to the nineteenth-century English workhouse, or poorhouse, transposed onto the social cartography of Canada by institutional practice and popular mythology. Although there was no physical structure called "The Poorhouse" in British Columbia, as there was in central and eastern parts of the country, old men and women still equated public facilities for the aged with that dreaded institution. Even today, some elderly Victoria residents speak of the Old Men's Home, closed nearly thirty years ago, in tones of dread and horror. Interviewed in 1990, Dr J. MacPherson, a dentist who visited the home as a young practitioner, said that these facilities were "sad places" and that "conditions were dreadful, yes, terrible."[4] As historian Michael Katz notes, a profound connection between old age homes, poverty, and death has remained in the public mind.[5]

This book takes the reader from the initial construction of homes for the aged in B.C. during the 1890s through to the 1960s, when federal and municipal involvement in the funding and provision of nursing home care was increasing. Overall, I present the Canadian old age home as an evolving institution, undergoing a fundamental shift from poor law facility to middle-class medical institution. Class, professionalism, and gender intersected in this progression. The cultural legacy of England's Poor Law, brought to Canada by British immigrants, transmitted from one generation to another, and reconfigured in various state and institutional policies and practices, is a theme that runs throughout this book. Canadians tend to view our modern health and welfare state as a national treasure, built in the post-Second World War era on the inspiration of progressive liberal figures such as Leonard Marsh and William Beveridge. But this system of governance did not spring forth like the first snowdrops after a cold winter. Rather, the welfare state created in the 1950s and 1960s was laid on top of older poor law institutions and programs. My appreciation of the historical provenance of state provision for old people and its institutional ramifications is based on the work of British historians Gertrude Himmelfarb, Geoffrey Finlayson, and Anne Crowther, and on Michael Katz's thoughtful American study of marginalized social groups.[6] In the Canadian contest, James Struther's excellent work on the history of state welfare has likewise been invaluable.[7]

The poor law is both theory and praxis, and the long historical shadow that it has cast over residential facilities for the aged requires an understanding of the workings of this early British system of welfare. A general increase in the numbers of indigent in Elizabethan times meant that the monasteries, the traditional source of poor relief, could no longer provide sufficient assistance, and in 1601 the state legislated the Poor Law. The parish became the basic unit of administration: a compulsory "poor rate" or tax was levied and distributed amongst the aged, sick, and poor by an overseer. Recipients could be paid in money or in kind, or they could be recruited for labour. The act divided the poor into two categories. Those seen as "deserving" of social support included the elderly, children, the infirm, and families in temporary difficulties. Migrant workers and beggars, considered "undeserving," were to be treated harshly. The former group were by law to be sent to the local workhouse for "indoor relief," but in fact usually received outdoor relief from the parish overseer. The latter were to be sent to a house of correction or house of industry, where they would work in exchange for a basic diet.

Changes brought about by the Industrial Revolution, including the devopment of large urban areas, a rapid population increase, and higher unemployment and food prices, led to increases in the poor rate, and in response to complaints from taxpayers the government enacted the New Poor Law of 1834. Intended to reduce costs, the New Poor Law instituted one poor relief system for England and Wales, created new administrative structures, built large workhouses, and established the key principle of "less eligibility." The concept of "less eligibility" meant that state aid was made as unattractive and minimal as possible, thereby forcing people to seek employment of any sort or help from family or friends before they turned to the state. Under this new system the old division between "deserving" and "undeserving" was rendered meaningless: old people and children were to be treated in the same punitive manner as migrants and beggars. Poorhouses, into which the aged were compelled to enter and were unlikely to be able to leave, were designed to be profoundly disempowering and humiliating, and their inmates led a wretched existence. Aged couples were separated, as men, women, and children were housed in different blocks; visiting hours between family members were restricted. Characteristics of the poorhouse included strict rules governing behaviour and social interaction and a requirement that inmates work for food and shelter. In this construct, state assistance is meant to be a demeaning, humbling, and depersonalizing experience, whether or not aid is given in the community or in a residential care facility. Thus enshrined within the culture of British public assistance programs, these parsimonious and harshly judgmental facets of the New Poor Law were deeply hated and sometimes violently opposed by the people whose lives they affected.

The principle of "less eligibility" was certainly a key factor in the management of workhouses in central and eastern Canada and, as my work demonstrates, the poor law has proved to be historically durable and exceptionally malleable. We need to comprehend the broad historical impact of the poor law on health and social assistance programs across the sweep of Canada's geographical and jurisdictional archipelago. I argue that the poor law was – and to a degree still is – a strong presence in B.C.'s old age homes. These places were not workhouses in the strict definition of the term, but administrative practices and cultural nuances common to them were derived from these earlier institutions. Thus it is no coincidence that early residents at B.C.'s provincial home for old men were denied the franchise: by entering what was essentially a poor law institution they automatically became less than full citizens.[8] Moreover, potential residents clearly regarded public institutions for the elderly through the cultural lens of the poor law, seeing them as a shameful place to end a life. Throughout this book, therefore, I evoke the poor law to help us appreciate the profound judgment and the power imbalance implicit in the culture of the old age home and present in many practices common to these facilities. There is a strong historical continuity in this regard.

The poor law ethos of need and right is often mediated by the special circumstances of the aged poor. Old people became destitute not because they were unwilling to work but because of age and ill health. Elderly inmates who ended up in the workhouse infirmary, a sector of the workhouse system for the chronically ill, were obviously too frail to labour for their keep. In B.C., I found a clearly identifiable group of economically and socially vulnerable single old men, cast-offs of the province's resource industries. Those who created and implemented health and social welfare policy were clearly aware of the precarious circumstances of this group. Moreover, there was a genuine appreciation for the fact that many "deserving" elderly indigents had been early pioneers of the coastal province. Social welfare discourse thus incorporated the concept of the "worthy pioneer," linked to the historical establishment of white British Columbia but now old and in need. Generally speaking, the public old age home in B.C. appears to have been a kinder, more benevolent place than in Ontario and the Maritime provinces. In this fashion poor law practices in British Columbia were tempered by a paternalistic sensitivity that was another characteristic of early welfare policy toward the aged, both within and without the institution. I see this paternalism as another thread that runs through the historical weave of welfare policy for the elderly, re-emerging under the welfare state in the practice of professional social workers and disappearing under the force of cost-cutting fiscal policy.

The institutional development of old age homes in Canada was also shaped by the jurisdictional responsibilities for health care and welfare provision set out in the 1867 British North America Act, which created the federal state of Canada. Under the act health care and social welfare fell under provincial jurisdiction, with the assumption being that welfare would be passed on to the municipal level of government. The development of institutions for the aged throughout the nineteenth century varied according to region, population growth, and rates of urbanization.[9] A Montreal workhouse was incorporated in 1818 and supported by grants from the legislature of Lower Canada. Similar institutions were established at Toronto in 1837 and in Kingston during the next decade.[10] The Protestant Home for the Aged (Men) and the Refuge Branch for Indigent and Aged Women were established in Ottawa in 1886 and 1888. Rural poorhouses were set up throughout Ontario during the 1860s and 1870s, while in Nova Scotia rural counties did not establish poorhouses until the final two decades of the century.[11]

During the late nineteenth century local almshouses in Britain and the United States began to be transformed into old age homes as children, the mentally ill, and others were relocated into specialized institutions.[12] In this analysis the twentieth-century old age home is presented as the reconstituted workhouse of a previous era. Anne Crowther and Michael Katz both see the poorhouse as a transitional institution from outdoor relief and the general workhouse to residential care for the aged.[13] This happened in some parts of Canada as well, although the pattern of change is not so tidy. By 1900 only the aged, the sick, and the "feeble-minded" were left in Ontario's Wellington County House of Industry.[14] In Nova Scotia, however, while the elderly comprised the majority of the institutional population, children, unwed mothers, and the "harmless insane" still resided in Halifax and district poorhouses well into the twentieth century.[15] This Maritime pattern and the evidence that I found in B.C. suggest that we need to conceptualize health and social welfare institutions as fluid constructs that respond as readily to need as to a prescribed clientele. I suspect that impoverished elderly people, especially women, were also regularly committed to B.C.'s provincial mental health facilities in the absence of any other place for them to live. It would be interesting to survey prison populations in the same light.

As my research evolved, I came to see health and welfare professionals as key in determining the shape that old age homes took during the twentieth century. These people, and the revisioned old age home that they strove to create, are best described as middle class. This is a problematic term in twentieth-century Canadian society, but it is useful for underscoring the sociological distance that often existed between professionals and their clients. Describing the new post-Second World

War old age home as middle class also helps us appreciate the way in which the institution and its perceived clientele were reinterpreted in this key period in the construction of the Canadian welfare state. My understanding of professionalism, bureaucracies, and policy development has been greatly advanced by the work of Harold Perkin, Theda Skocpol, Linda Gordon, and James Struthers.[16] Policy formation needs to be understood as a complex, multi-faceted process, with input taking place at three levels. Politicians and senior civil servants shape policy in its initial stages, often relying on information gathered by academics or other policy specialists. The resulting programs are reshaped at the service level both by those delivering care and by those receiving care. In terms of institutions, notions about the senescence were also reflected in the architecture of old age homes and in the way in which interior space was organized and decorated.

This book goes beyond an analysis of the cultural and political place of the old age home to look at the elderly men and women who entered its doors. This social history is rooted in my own life history. Like many young women who grew up in the retirement community of Victoria, I found casual employment in my late teens and early twenties with the elderly. Criss-crossing town on a borrowed bicycle, I worked as a homemaker for old people, cleaning immaculate apartments, chatting, and eating Peak Frean cookies. My personal life during this period intersected with aged kin as well. I witnessed my grandfather's struggle with his wife's worsening mental and physical health, then mourned his own death. Digging into my great-aunt's pension surplus, rapidly accumulating while she remained in an extended care unit, my mother and I took her on wild and luxurious sprees to the Calgary Palliser and the Vancouver Hyatt-Regency Hotels. When she broke her hip in the summer of 1988, I held her hand all afternoon and evening in the hospital; the staff finally acquiesced to our combined tenacity and allowed her to wear her cherished wedding rings in surgery.

I do not believe we should romanticize the elderly, and I could rewrite this last paragraph to set the aging men and women whose lives were part of mine in a negative, unappealing light. But my point is that my time with old people taught me invaluable lessons about the survival strategies of the elderly and the way in which health, money, and sociability set boundaries on their daily lives. I grew to comprehend the very gendered nature of the culture of old age. I also came to appreciate the profound courage and dignity of the aged. These personal experiences are the ghost behind the social history in this volume. As an historian, I want to introduce you to old people of the past. I want my reader to put on the shoes of the elderly, sit in their place, and live alongside them in their home and in the institution.

This goal is more radical than it might seem at first, for western society is deeply ageist.[17] It is not so much that we see old people as deviant as that we do not see them at all. Ageism is pervasive within academia as well. Despite the flowering of Canadian social history in the last three decades, which in turn has sparked interest in educational history, women's history, labour history, urban history, and gender history, there has been little work on the lives of old people. Most Canadian historians may have accepted the importance of gender, class, and race, but we need to learn to apply the category of age in a consistent analytical fashion as well.

This book, then, writes older men and women into the historical record, examining their lives and survival strategies as they sought to live independently outside the old age home. On a theoretical level, the first chapter is very much informed by the rich body of historical literature that employs the life cycle approach. The work of Tamara Hareven and Michael Anderson, as well as many others, has been particularly useful, allowing me to play off B.C.'s large population of single, aging, labouring men against careful demographic studies of old people elsewhere in other periods.[18] Except where the names of individuals were already provided in published source material, I inserted pseudonyms that reflected the ethnic origins of the individual in question. Using pseudonyms is of course necessary in order to protect the privacy of individuals. I believe that my decision to give complete personal and family names helps the reader to see the people who inhabit these pages as human beings and thus honours the complexity of their lives and experiences.[19] Building particularly on James Snell's work on the lives of old people in Canada's past, I consider the factors that made elderly people vulnerable to institutionalization.[20]

My analysis of economic and practical strategies for independent living is based on the assumption that old people preferred to live in the community rather than in an institution. This perspective is based in part on my wish to present the elderly as active agents, but it is also strongly supported by other historians of old age working in a variety of time periods and geographical locations.[21] Certainly, my own research provides numerous illustrations of elderly women and men working hard to hold onto their cherished independence. Intellectually, I can appreciate the theories about the creation of structured dependency through the growth of welfare state programs and retirement legislation that have been so passionately argued by Chris Phillipson and others.[22] But in my heart I believe that old people were profoundly appreciative of the pension and that it really changed their lives for the better.

Race is as important as class and gender in the study of old age. In this book I bring in ethnicity where sources allow me to do so, highlighting the connection between ethnicity and B.C.'s particular population of single, aging men. I talk about Chinese, Italian, and Scandinavian older people, but I do not talk about elderly men and women from First Nations communities. This omission does not reflect my measure of the importance of First Nations people, for of course they still comprised about a quarter of B.C.'s population in the first years of this study. Rather, this is due to the almost complete absence of this group from my data – by the 1940s only a handful of First Nations people had appeared among the institutional populations that I studied.

The fact that I did not "find" First Nations people among the residential populations that I considered is in part a reflection of my reliance on provincial and municipal archival sources. Yet this finding also raises a number of interesting questions. With an equal gender population profile and stronger traditions of family and community, were First Nations communities simply better at caring for their aged? Historians have rightly seen First Nations people as the focus of white medical imperialism, but did their exclusion from the mandate of B.C.'s dynamic provincial health and welfare state of the 1930s mean that their elders escaped the professional appropriation that I describe in chapter 3 of this book? Did their absence from municipal relief rolls mean that they were not forced to enter the despised public old age home? Without doubt, First Nations people's cultural understanding of the old age home would have been shaped by the residential school experience rather than by the English Poor Law.

In short, I speculate that the experience of older First Nations people was very different than other groups in Canadian society up until the 1940s. My suspicion is that this cohort, along with many others of that community, were drawn into the reconfigured institutional scene following the Second World War – perhaps becoming patients in the burgeoning geriatric psychiatric facilities that mushroomed in discarded military facilities in B.C.'s hinterlands. But that story, important as it may be, is not the focus of this book.

How likely were British Columbia's elders to end their lives in a residential care institution? This is a difficult question to answer. David Thomson found that the institutionalization of elderly men and women in England has followed a wave pattern over the past two centuries, peaking in 1900, dropping over the first decades of the twentieth century, and then rising again during the 1950s.[23] The population of B.C.'s old age homes clearly expanded during the period that I consider, although my calculations cannot be exact.[24] In the early 1930s there were some 300 men and women over the age of sixty-five in charitable and benevolent institutions in the province and another

300 beds in private hospitals that cared for adults.[25] In 1941 there were 954 spaces in charitable and benevolent facilities and another 592 beds in private nursing homes that specialized in chronic illness and convalescent care.[26] By 1957, the final year for which statistics are available for private hospitals in B.C., there were 1,740 beds in the latter category alone.[27] For 1931 and 1941, the institutional statistics represent some 1.6 and 2.3 per cent of the total number of people in B.C. over sixty-five years of age.

Other data also points to the widening use of old age homes. The number of provincially licensed charitable and benevolent homes for "infirm or unemployable adults," an administrative category that referred almost exclusively to the aged, increased from 68 in 1948 to 120 in 1951.[28] By 1953 Edith Pringle, provincial inspector of hospitals, was describing British Columbians as being "almost wholly dependent upon the service now being rendered by privately operated hospitals or so-called nursing homes."[29]

But statistics tell only part of the story. In this book I take the reader inside the cultural and material world of residential care facilities. This allows us to measure new professional ideals against methods of governance at work within the old age home. I draw deeply here on the work of Erving Goffman and other social control theorists who have studied contemporary old age homes. The Canadian old age home needs to be understood as an instrument of social control so that we can comprehend both the differential possession of power in the lives of the poor and disadvantaged and some of the unique characteristics of the institutional world. I was fortunate to be able to draw on a considerable body of Canadian research into the history of workhouses and public homes for the aged. My own work on this topic has been strengthened by the scholarship of Stormi Stewart, James Snell, James Struthers, and Edgar-André Montigny.[30] Elizabeth Janeway's superb analysis on the subject of power relations and my own personal and professional experiences with the elderly, mental health patients, and young children have sharpened my understanding of discontent and rebellion among the disempowered.[31] Peter Townsend's seminal work *The Last Refuge* is a classic and powerful statement on behalf of old people.[32]

I deal with a number of different institutions in this book, some of which I revisit in various contexts. Over the period the provincial government operated the Provincial Home for Aged Men in Kamloops and established a Provincial Infirmary system, a network of old age homes for the chronically ill and disabled that included the Home for Incurables (later renamed the Provincial Infirmary at Marpole) in Vancouver, Mount Saint Mary's in Victoria, and the Allco Infirmary in the Fraser

Valley. The City of Victoria ran the Old Men's Home and the City of Vancouver operated the Old People's Home (later Taylor Manor). The first philanthropic homes for the elderly included the Home for Aged and Infirm Ladies (now known as Rose Manor) and the Zhonghua Yiyuan (Chinese Hospital), both located in Victoria. Philanthropic old age homes rapidly expanded in the post-Second World War period, as did municipal facilities. I discuss a considerable number of these later institutions, including the Victoria Nursing Home (Gorge Road Hospital), Prince Rupert's Pioneer Home, Kelowna's David Lloyd-Jones Home, and the Salvation Army's Matson Lodge in Victoria.

The chapter organization was conceived as a way of taking my reader through a journey of the senescence. I begin with a chapter about the elderly in the community, to illuminate both the factors that made old people vulnerable to institutionalization and the strategies that they used to hold onto their independence. The second chapter puts the facilities whose gates they might have entered into the frame, tracing the institutional evolution of different old age homes in B.C. Chapter 3 discusses changing ideas and ideals of institutional provision for the aged, giving a cultural dimension to the bricks and mortar presented in chapter 2. The fourth chapter takes the reader inside the world of the institution to present a picture of patient life. And the final chapter considers the place of the old age home within the emerging welfare state, applying broader questions about community and institutional care to an innovative program of the 1930s that sought to de-institutionalize B.C.'s aged.

This volume covers a broad chronological sweep in the history of British Columbia. In 1891, when this study begins, the province was only twenty years old, with an estimated population of 27,305 First Nations peoples and 70,865 non-aboriginals. Among this latter group, only 25 per cent were women and fewer than 2.5 per cent were over the age of sixty-five – a small irony given today's image of B.C. as a haven for retirees. By 1961 this demographic profile had entirely altered, with a total population of 1,092,099 and roughly even numbers of women and men. Historically, B.C.'s economic base has been built on its primary resources – fish, timber, and minerals – throughout the province, while the majority of the population clustered around Vancouver and Victoria. Settlement patterns and economic factors had a significant impact on health and social welfare systems, fostering strong provincial involvement and a weak municipal base in the provision of services in these sectors.[33]

Although my study of the history of elderly people and old age homes in Canada is set in British Columbia, the broad themes of the book have a national resonance. The shift from poor law facility to middle-class medical institution happened all across the country, although the limited amount of research that has been done suggests that pace varied according to region.[34] The new post-war architecture of the old age home and the efforts to "re-form" the institution through renaming and redecoration clearly had an impact in the prairies and the central region. Federal initiatives, from the Old Age Pension Act of 1927 to the 1957 Hospital Diagnostics Act, also helped reshape the economics of the Canadian old age home. A handful of critical elements of this study transcend national boundaries: the ever-increasing demand for residential care for old people, the efforts of elderly men and women to remain living independently in old age, and the importance of family, community, and pensions in the strategies that they adopted.

But the greatest commonality between old age homes in B.C. and elsewhere was the cultural place of the poorhouse. Statistically, the chances of an old person entering an institution like Vancouver's Old People's Home were small. But, as those who study residential care facilities today note, the fear of institutionalization is strong among *all* aged people.[35] Within the walls of the old age home in the western province the culture of the poorhouse prevailed. This was not a regional phenomenon but part of the baggage of the British Poor Laws, which immigrated to Canada along with the British people.

To understand the cultural space that the old age home occupies in Canadian society today, we must appreciate this ethos in the context of what it is to grow old and look into the face of poverty, infirmity, and death. This is a feeling and an experience, not a statistic. There is a vast silence about the essence of the old age home, both in the past and in the present, yet this is not because there is no tale to be told.[36] I believe this book needs to be read, not just for its data and analysis, but because it offers an historical hinge between our own lives and the house of old.

1 Before the Institution: Coping Strategies and Vulnerability

The struggle for self is a primal drama of old age. In our youth we quest to gain power, we bargain and fight to define who we are. In our middle years we seek to find ourselves in work and in the emotional worlds of partnership and parenting. In the last decades we no longer quest, but hold tight to personal autonomy garnered over the span of a lifetime. The diminution of the self, and the passage into the house of old, takes many shapes. It can be swift: a broken hip, a severe stroke, the death of a spouse. Or it can be a longer process, a measured awareness of physical and material losses: the trip to the store now too far to undertake, the cobwebs behind the toilet now ignored.

The men and women whose lives are at the heart of this book looked institutionalization right in the face – and they did not like what they saw. Many hated the idea of a residential facility, sometimes waging battle against kin, community, and the state as they held tight to their independence. The elderly of British Columbia from the 1890s to the 1960s, like aged people in other locales and time periods, placed a high value on personal autonomy and worked hard to stay outside the old age home.[1] They strategized, using personal assets, good health, casual labour, and help from spouses, neighbours, offspring, and the state. Old age pensions, introduced in B.C. in 1927, rapidly became an important aid to independent living in senescence. If money, home, and health remained in good balance, then an older man or woman could continue to live independently. But if one element in this often fragile equation fell apart, then they might well be forced to enter an old age home.

The experience of old age was sharply defined by marital status, gender, community, ethnicity, and class. Support from spouses and children was often critical for elderly men and women. Old women were more likely to receive help from kin, assistance sometimes denied to male relations. Savings, pensions, and property helped ensure financial stability in old age. Neighbours and ethnic communities were another resource for those growing old and infirm.

Historically, the last stage of the life cycle has been characterized by deprivation among those on the economic margins.[2] The aged poor have always suffered hardship, but old people without family occupy a particularly precarious position. Unlike rural Ontario, British Columbia did not have settled agrarian communities with established traditions of supporting aged kin.[3] Instead, the dominance of resource-based industries meant that British Columbia had a significant population of elderly single labouring men, many of whom had been transient workers in their young and middle years. This is a different historical pattern than that found in other locations in the western world, where elderly females living alone outnumbered single old men. The extreme marginalization of B.C.'s elderly working-class bachelors shows us that until the 1950s there was a unique kind of underclass in the province, aged and impoverished cast-offs of resource capitalism.[4] The pattern of their last years was still male-centred, migratory, and constructed outside a mainstream society that increasingly perceived the middle-class family as the norm.

I did not want to try and push the data presented in this chapter into a definitive chronology. With the obvious and important exception of the introduction of old age pensions, change was too diffuse and individual circumstances too diverse for me to be certain that I was charting explicit shifts. Instead, I chose to consider strategies and situations, looking at how old people lived from the vantage point of the aged themselves and of their kin and community. I am interested in the world of old age, in uncovering the agency of elderly men and women, and in the ways that other people and community structures gave assistance. The old people whose stories I tell were those most vulnerable to institutionalization – working people on the margins, the infirm elderly, widows, men without family. This is not a chapter about the middle-class elderly in British Columbia. I begin by looking at specific populations of elders in B.C. – single and working men, women, and people with partners and family – and assessing their strategies in old age. I then turn to an analysis of how community and state assistance worked to support the aged living outside institutions.

MEN WITHOUT FAMILIES

Most historians of old age have studied the elderly who live in long-established communities with a settled workforce, a network of

Table 1
Number of males per 100 females, selected provinces, 1901–1951

	1901	1911	1921	1931	1941	1951
British Columbia	177	179	127	125	114	105
Alberta	128	149	123	121	115	110
Manitoba	119	121	111	111	108	103
Ontario	101	106	102	104	103	101
Nova Scotia	103	104	104	105	105	102

Source: 1951 census, table 20.

intergenerational families, and equal populations of men and women. The historical demography of old age in Canada, however, must be mapped out with an appreciation for settlement and generational patterns and for the economic opportunities offered by different geographical settings. From 1891 to 1951 the provincial population profiles of central and eastern Canada show a mature population with balanced gender ratios at all stages of the life cycle, a picture that obscures the existence of male-dominated resource communities in northern Ontario and Quebec. In the prairie provinces of Manitoba and Saskatchewan the shift toward a gender-balanced population indicates the progression from the beginnings of non-aboriginal settlement to the family farm. As family settlement increased, the demographic profile grew to resemble that of Ontario and Nova Scotia.

There was a different pattern in the western and northern regions of the country. The historical demography of B.C., Alberta, and the Northwest and Yukon Territories reveals a gender imbalance that continued well into the twentieth century: as was the case in New Zealand in the first decades following sustained settlement,[5] non-aboriginal men significantly outnumbered women at all stages of the adult life cycle.[6] In 1901 there were 177 men to every 100 women in B.C., a much larger proportion than in Alberta and other provinces. In succeeding decades Alberta and B.C.'s gender ratios became more similar – a reflection of the growth of cattle ranching in Alberta – but the gap between men and women remained larger in B.C., a demographic characteristic of a settler society, which it retained until the 1940s.

Taking the population of the province as a whole, the gender imbalance in B.C. had disappeared by 1950. However, as might be expected, the early influx of men remained and many grew old without marrying. Table 2 shows that men continued to dominate the elderly population of B.C. even when the province was becoming a popular retirement destination. Until the 1961 census, men over sixty-five years of age

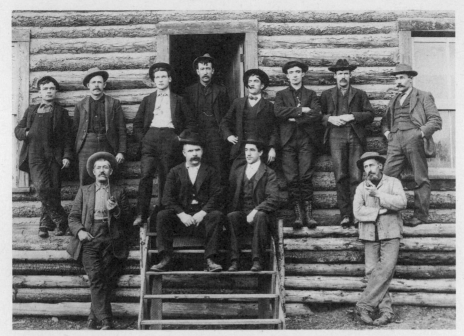

Men at Camp McKinney, Cariboo Region, 1900s. This group of B.C. miners demonstrates the demographic dominance of men in the early years of European settlement. Many of these men, unskilled, single, and transient throughout their lives, would become vulnerable to poverty and institutionalization in their last years. (British Columbia Provincial Archives)

Table 2
Number of men per 100 women
in the population over 65 years of age,
Canada and B.C., 1901–1961

	Canada	B.C.
1901	81	174
1921	105	138
1941	104	133
1961	94	104

Source: Censuses of Canada, 1901–1961

were more numerous than their female cohorts.[7] Within this group of older males were the never-married men who had come in their youth to work in B.C.'s resource-based industries. Peter Ward refers to this cohort when he notes that by 1941 B.C.'s demographic profile looked more like the rest of Canada because of the "gradual ageing and death of the remaining surplus male population."[8]

Instead of the family farm, the basis for agrarian settlement in the rest of western Canada, much of B.C. had the logging or mining camp, where women and children were a relative novelty. Young men provided the labour in isolated and impermanent resource-based communities, and immigrant labourers from continental Europe and Asia formed a sizeable portion of this workforce. By 1900 Vancouver was the hub of economic life in B.C. and labouring men would typically migrate to that city, or perhaps Victoria, when employment was scarce or to escape the cold winters in the north or interior regions of the province.[9] Born in what is now Hungary around 1885, Leo Paulcer spent the 1930s and early 1940s prospecting and working in various B.C. fish canneries and logging and mining camps. The working men's hotels along Pender Street were his bases that he returned to between jobs.[10] Men like Paulcer were not family men, nor were such locales likely to foster the development of families and stable, intergenerational communities. Such workers were rarely able to accumulate the capital necessary to marry and establish a family.[11] This population cohort moved across the historical continuum of twentieth-century British Columbia, a generation of single men who faced old age with few financial resources, no family, and no secure place within a settled supportive community.

Male immigrants from continental Europe or Asia were most likely to be without kin in old age. Table 3 shows the "racial" origin of men and women resident in B.C. over fifty-five and sixty-five years of age in 1931, the only year when the census reported on age and race. Older men were numerically dominant in all categories but particularly among continental Europeans and Asians. Many of the old men who surfaced for the 1931 census would also have been counted, as younger men, for the 1911 census, where men from central Europe, Italy, and Japan outnumbered women four to one. Scandinavian men also significantly outnumbered their womenfolk in 1911 and the female populations in the East Indian and Chinese communities were practically non-existent.

Typically, these single men from Europe and Asia emigrated to B.C. and found unskilled work on railway construction and in mines and canneries. The isolated places where they worked, the barriers created by language, and their single status kept them on the margins of B.C. society. Unlike their British cohorts, these single working men did not become part of a nuclear family as they moved through their adult years. Even Scandinavian men, the non-English-speaking immigrants most easily assimilated into mainstream North American society, were slow to marry and establish families in Canada.

In their heads and hearts many immigrant workers had only a temporary stake in British Columbia, never intending to grow old in a

Table 3
Number of men per 100 women (over 55 and 65 years
of age) according to ethnic and "racial" origin, B.C., 1931

Ethnicity/"Race"	55+	65+
British	133	128
Continental European	195	185
Asiatic	222	214
Indian	105	102

Source: Canadian censuses, 1931

foreign land. Many Italian workers returned each winter to their home-land.[12] Some Chinese men saved enough for a return trip to visit China and perhaps to marry there, but only a few managed to bring their wives and children to Canada.[13] Gender imbalance and the problems it created in old age were well recognized in the Chinese-Canadian community.[14] While the dream was always to return to China, many Chinese immigrants ended their lives alone in Canada. East Indian men, too, worked with the goal of accumulating family capital in the Punjab. After 1908, federal regulations made it virtually impossible for East Indian men to bring their wives and children to Canada.[15]

The large number of single men in the province meant that many men could not count on two traditional caregivers, wives and female children, to sustain them as they grew older. Unmarried and widowed men were typically over-represented in workhouses across the United States, in Britain, and in other parts of Canada during the late nineteenth and early twentieth centuries,[16] but it is the aging single men of New Zealand that bear the strongest similarity to their British Columbian brothers.[17] Lack of kin made B.C.'s aging loggers, prospectors, miners, and fishers particularly vulnerable to destitution, homelessness, and institutionalization. The records of the provincial Indigent Fund, the only public source of income support for old people living outside municipal boundaries in the late nineteenth and early twentieth century, are filled with reports of poverty-stricken old men without family. Inmate registers at the Provincial Home for Aged Men show a very high proportion of unmarried residents: the percentage of single men ranged from 70 per cent in the period between 1900 and 1916 to 55 per cent in the period between 1949 and 1951.[18] Patient statistics compiled in 1945 at Vancouver's Marpole branch of the Provincial Infirmary, an adult facility for the physically disabled, show that 67 per cent of its male residents over the age of sixty had never been married or were separated from their spouses.[19]

Dislocation from family is striking in the personal histories of male inmates in B.C.'s public institutions. Not only were these men unable

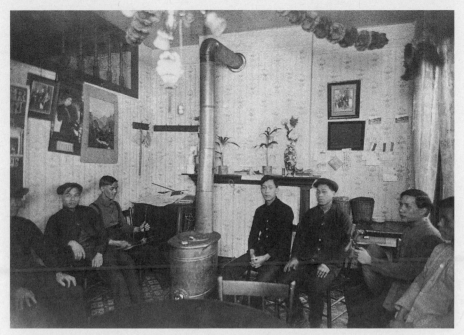

Men in a rooming house, Chinatown, Vancouver, 1902. Men in ethnic groups where
women were very few in number were particularly vulnerable when they grew older.
Gender imbalance and the problems it created in old age were well recognized in
the Chinese-Canadian community, which established care facilities for their aged
compatriots in Victoria and Vancouver during the late nineteenth century. (British
Columbia Provincial Archives)

to establish their own nuclear families during their young and middle
years but they often lost touch with sisters, brothers, and parents when
they migrated west. A woman in Montana, informed in 1925 of her
brother's death at the Provincial Home, replied that she had not seen
her brother since she was a young girl and knew little about his life.[20]
John Duffy, a single Irish labourer who applied for assistance in
Vancouver in 1907, had long since lost contact with relatives left
behind in Ireland and Toronto.[21] Lost and distant families were of little
help when an old man grew ill or could not find work.

Patterns in old age mirrored those of the younger and middle years
of the life cycle, but with a heightened risk of ill health, poverty, and
homelessness. Because they had not made the transition to marriage,
nor set down roots in one location, these men did not have the community standing that marriage and family life brought.[22] Nor is it
likely that they had the social refinements of speech and manner
expected in "respectable" working-class or middle-class society:
camp life is depicted by Martin Grainger and others as aggressively

masculine, characterized by hard drinking and rough language.[23] To the degree that these men were socially accepted, it was as "boys," irresponsible men who lived outside society's boundaries (both literally and figuratively) and had never grown up enough to take on the full responsibilities of citizenship and family life.[24]

Many older unmarried labouring men like John Duffy continued to follow a transient life pattern as they aged, spending summers on the road and taking shelter in urban communities when the weather turned cold. Eighty-four-year-old Ian Gray, interviewed by a provincial government agent in 1925, had been a miner and prospector. Nine months of the year were spent away from urban centres, but he returned each winter to live in a Vernon hotel.[25] Another pensioner described his seasonal migrations in the 1940s: "Every year I leave Vancouver on March 1st for Hope – then I have a tent and camp on the Coquihalla River for 2 months, then I go to Princeton and camp on 9 Mile Creek – 9 miles west of Princeton for 2 months – then I walk over the Dewdney trail to Hope and camp there till the end of October – I then leave for Vancouver for the winter."[26] Such a survival strategy clearly depended on good health.[27]

There was continuity between youth and old age in the life cycles of these men. Many aging men without family made their way to a familiar urban area where relief could be obtained, friends could be found, and cheap housing was available. The life experience of these old bachelors – who had typically spent their youth in Europe, emigrated across the Atlantic, laboured in remote regions of Canada and the United States, and perhaps been involved in radical politics – meant that their urban communities were often cosmopolitan and multi-ethnic. Leo Paulcer, for example, who lived in a Vancouver rooming house in 1949, had journeyed from Hungary to Hamburg to New York, worked in various mining operations across the United States and into B.C. from 1903 until 1944, and been a member of the Industrial Workers of the World.[28]

In Victoria, aging men found accommodation at the Salvation Army Hostel, in a row of cabins on Pembroke Street, or at rooming houses and hotels such as the Clifton Rooms or the Ritz Hotel.[29] The temperate weather of the southern coastal towns was attractive to many old men, although some preferred the drier air of the Kamloops area as it helped alleviate miners' consumption.[30]

Elderly male labourers who came to Vancouver lived in brick rooming houses or pensioner's hotels along Pender Street and on the edge of the working-class Strathcona district. Some lived in "coolie cabins," bunkhouse structures with narrow external porches and small single rooms clustered in Vancouver's waterfront area. In 1912 municipal health officials looked at sixty-two of these cabins and described them

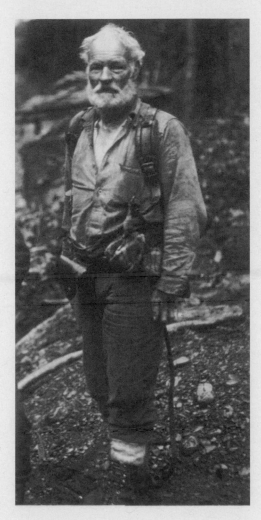

"The Prospector," near Vancouver, 1920. This image of a prospector evokes the romantic qualities of these men that so appealed to provincial social workers of the 1940s and 1950s. Independent, resourceful, and a direct link with B.C.'s pioneer past, such clients were thought to need help from modern health and welfare professionals to deal with social problems in old age. (Percy Bentley, F.R.P.S.)

as dirty, poorly lit, and lacking proper ventilation.[32] However, the cabins remained favourite homes for retired labouring men. Here old bachelors like Pat Fitzpatrick, an Irish immigrant who had spent a life working on B.C.'s railroads, baked sourdough bread, split his own wood, and cooked mutton stew. For Fitzpatrick and his neighbours, this accommodation offered independence and privacy in old age.[33]

Aging men also congregated in Vancouver's Hastings Street area, undoubtedly recalling the neighbourhood's "bar rooms, cafes, pool halls, second-hand stores and boarding-houses" from when they had come to

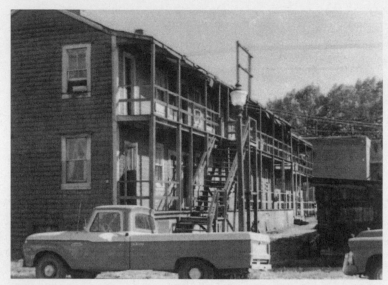

The last of the "coolie cabins," East Vancouver, 1972. Condemmed by municipal health officals as early as 1912 as dirty, ill-lit, and lacking proper ventilation, these frame bunkhouses, clustered in Vancouver's waterfront area, remained popular homes for retired labouring men. (Rolf Knight, private collection)

the city as young labourers. Their days were spent in the local area, drinking coffee in the White Lunch diner, hanging around Victory Square, or visiting the Universal Bookstore on East Hastings. These places, like similar establishments in Victoria and elsewhere, were set apart from the wider context of working-class culture by the fact that these men had once been employed in the woods, mines, and fisheries of the province. The urban spaces used by these men were quite distinct from parts of the city where middle- and working-class families lived. As Martin Grainger notes in *Woodsmen of the West*, this was male urban territory.[31]

Ethnicity and racism created separate urban enclaves for old men. In Victoria and Vancouver's Chinatowns single old men were part of the larger community of Chinese men. Like their younger male coun- trymen, elderly Chinese men lived in small rooms in wooden boarding houses, back-alley shacks, and shop cellars. Usually they would cook, live, and sleep in one room, often sharing the space with roommates.[34]

Geographically, in both cities the elderly single European men and their Chinese counterparts lived only a few blocks apart. Socially, their worlds were totally separate. By the late 1920s and 1930s, because of the new Chinese Immigration Act, B.C.'s Chinatowns were aging,

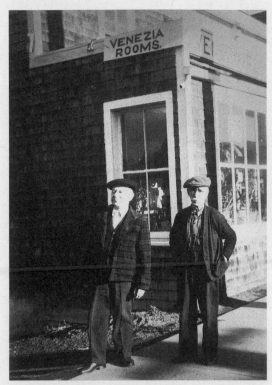

Two men outside the Venezia Rooms, Kamloops, 1911.
This 1911 image shows two older men outside what may
have been their rooming house. Many aging working
men without families moved into the urban settings that
they were familiar from their earlier years, cobbling
together money from odd jobs, savings, and pension
funds to survive. (British Columbia Provincial Archives)

growing smaller, and turning inward.[35] Not all Chinese men, of course,
lived in urban centres: in 1925 the government agent in Smithers
reported that a penniless Chinese miner was being supported by aboriginal people at Fort Babine.[36] Phyllis and Ali Knight gave their Lillooet
cabin to an old and nearly blind Chinese prospector a decade later.[37]

Other men who had never married lived alone in remote shacks in
the woodlands or mountains of rural British Columbia, places where
they had spent their working lives.[38] As James Snell notes, we cannot
be sure how many older men lived in this fashion, taking care of their
limited material needs by trapping, prospecting or "scrounging."[39]
Seventy-two-year-old Bjorn Sondstrom, living in Sirdar in 1925, paid
no rent for his shack and had a boat that he used to catch fish. This

was, he maintained, much better than living in the Provincial Home.[40] Businesses sometimes allowed old men to take shelter in unused buildings, like the Frenchman who lived in a cabin on Canadian Collieries property near Nanaimo in 1924.[41]

Some older single men had houses on land that was their own. Bachelors who had managed to acquire property were well served by their investment in old age, as it brought a degree of financial security and enabled them to hold onto their independence for longer than those without houses and land. If a bachelor was also integrated into the local community, which was more likely in small towns and farming settlements, then he might get help from his neighbours in times of crisis. Men in this situation were not perceived or treated as marginal: ownership of a home gave them an acknowledged place within the local community. The stories of three men illustrate how property helped ensure autonomy. Robert Marland, an elderly bachelor farmer, cultivated enough vegetables for his own use on his two-acre plot of land in the farming and logging district of Beaver Point on Saltspring Island at the close of World War One. His long membership in the small group of local settlers – and status as one of the original preemptors in the area – meant that he received financial and practical help when he grew ill.[42] Ownership of property clearly allowed Marland self-sufficiency and community support as he grew old.

The theme of self-sufficiency is strong in the tales of the other two men as well, showing how property could produce much needed supplements to limited retirement savings or pension payments. Matthew Barker was a seventy-six-year-old bachelor who lived near Vernon during the 1940s in what was described as "typical hermit's quarters." This residence, where the "old dog, favourite chickens and rabbits wander in and out at will," did not meet the standards of the local social worker. Nonetheless, the reference to poultry suggests a measure of self-sufficiency, and it is clear that Barker, a former butcher, lumberjack, and fireman, was quite content with his home.[43] Similarly, a retired Norwegian who had spent a lifetime fishing off the northern coast of British Columbia built a cabin on a local island in 1950 and lived there comfortably for four years, "obtaining a good deal of his food from natural sources."[44]

In their youth B.C.'s transient working men, the larger-than-life heroes of Martin Grainger's *Woodsmen of the West*, were symbols of the province's early history of resource extraction and capital exploitation.[45] As they grew old, they used coping strategies and locales from their young and middle years in their bid to remain independent. Old age mirrored youth in the migratory patterns of unmarried working men, in the use of urban working-class boarding houses and hotels, and in the experience of economic uncertainty. The aging bachelor logger or miner was not a ready fit for twentieth-century British Columbia society, with its dream of single family dwellings in green suburbs and small towns. As Robert McDonald points out, class, race, ethnicity, and masculinity worked together to shut these single men off from the "respectable" community of married men and women.[46] Their lack of kinship networks made them especially prone to impoverishment and institutionalization. The alternative male culture of old age in which these men participated continued to be a part of B.C.'s urban, working-class landscape and a feature of rural areas of the province well into the 1950s.

OLD MEN AND WAGED LABOUR

For older working-class men in late nineteenth- and early twentieth-century British Columbia, earning an income was a critical part of their strategy for remaining independent.[47] Retirement, one of the grand social projects of the twentieth century, was simply not an option for working people,[48] and this remained the case even after the introduction of old age pensions, for the payments did not fully cover the cost of living, and the limited criteria for eligibility excluded many old people. The ability of men to hold onto viable employment, however, weakened as they aged. The men whose lives are chronicled here were those who ended their days in need, receiving state assistance or entering a public old age home. Their stories illustrate how the structure of B.C.'s economy created a group of vulnerable, impoverished old men.

Although retirement was becoming increasingly accepted in Canada by the 1940s, the term did not apply to most men who were forced to enter public facilities. Those applying to Victoria's Old Men's Home commonly used phrases such as "I am too old to work," or "I am sick"; few described themselves as "retired." Uncertain personal finances and a life structured around work meant that working-class men, both single and married, worked as long as they physically could. This interpretation is supported by American data collected by Howard Chudacoff and Tamara Hareven, who found that 60 per cent of men over sixty-five were still working in the 1920s and 1930s.[49] The older men whom I am looking at were shifting downward in the labour market in terms of status and pay, rather than out of waged work entirely.

Middle-class clerks or professionals and skilled craftsmen or agricultural workers – people who grew old in the workplace they had laboured in as younger men – fared better than did loggers, miners, and other unskilled labourers. Men in trade, services, or financial sectors of the economy had the best opportunities for aging men: they were valued for the knowledge and skills that they in turn passed on to the next generation of workers, and as they aged they often remained in the same place but took on lighter, less financially remunerative tasks. They might be paid less and have a lower status, but a paternalistic system ensured a degree of financial stability in old age and ongoing inclusion in the male world of the workplace.[50]

The pattern of skilled or semi-skilled working men being pushed into unskilled labour as they aged that has been found elsewhere is evident in B.C.[51] Applicants to the Old Men's Home in Victoria who had been de-skilled in this fashion often gave two occupations – their craft and an unskilled job that they had followed "lately." Those who had been skilled workers when young, like the Smithers resident who had done carpentry and roof repairs,[52] became casual labourers as they grew older.

By far the largest category of men who entered old age homes, however, were unskilled labourers. Typically, such men had worked in their youth on railways and in mining and logging, in jobs for men with strong bodies and physical endurance. Census takers found that B.C. consistently had a higher percentage of men who declared themselves to be labourers than the national average.[53] As they grew older, loggers, miners, and fishers could not hope to hold onto the physically strenuous work of their youth. Moreover, the transient nature of the employment market meant that they would rarely have a long-standing relationship with one company that might be repaid by paternalism in old age.

Thus part of the difficulty that aging labouring men faced in B.C. was the youthful character of the labour market in the resource sector, yet in all areas of male employment earnings dropped and unemployment increased with age. Eric Sager and Peter Baskerville's analysis of the 1891 census for Vancouver, Victoria, and New Westminster revealed this pattern and found that the proportion of males who had no stated occupation increased with age, from 8.5 per cent of men in their fifties to 29.5 per cent of men in their seventies.[54] Their findings, based on urban data, only hint at the particular situation of older men in a resource-based economy.

The work patterns of older labouring men in B.C., then, bear a closer resemblance to those of urban industrial workers than to agricultural workers, their rural counterparts. Like the urban industrial labourer, the aging resource worker in B.C. was not so much de-skilled as entirely displaced.[55] The period in the male life cycle following middle age was one in which uncertain health and diminishing physical strength closed off employment possibilities. Shut out from former places of employment, these men could only find jobs that were poorly paid, fragmented, and low status. Work for aging loggers and miners was therefore entirely divorced from their former employment within the resource sector, creating two distinct phases to their working life. No gains in terms of skills or loyalty could be rewarded when one passed from one phase of the working life cycle to another.

What kinds of work did I find old men doing in B.C.? As elsewhere in Canada, aging males found irregular waged labour that was unskilled, light, poorly paid, and often seasonal.[56] Kindly Annie Larkin employed two elderly men to pull thistles in her Ganges garden on Saltspring Island.[57] A man on leave from the Old Men's Home in Kamloops picked berries in Naramata.[58] A sixty-four-year-old Victoria pensioner in the 1940s found work doing chores for a woman in the affluent Rockland area of the city. He was paid forty cents per hour.[59] The government agent in Cranbrook in 1926 reported the arrival of a Vancouver man in his seventies who was "going around the country sharpening lawn-mowers and scissors for a living."[60]

Old men felt the constraints of age and circumstance keenly. In 1919 one elderly man reported, "My sore knee, and deafness prevent me from competing with returned soldiers, and Orientals."[61] Placed with other marginal employables in a pool of unskilled labourers, old men moved in and out of waged labour as the market, rather than their needs, dictated. Returning soldiers and immigrants may have undermined the employment possibilities of old men in 1920, but the Great Depression decimated the employment market for aged people.[62] In contrast, the Second World War and the rising demand for labour created by Canada's war effort meant that aging men found new and expanded employment opportunities.

At least until the onset of the Depression, work on provincial and municipal roads that was less physically demanding was set aside for elderly male labourers – a traditional form of relief for old men in Britain.[63] Elderly men worked on the province's public highways during the summer months, like the Saltspring Island men who cleared brush from the roadsides.[64] An eighty-four-year-old bachelor interviewed in 1925 had spent the past seven years keeping the road between Vernon and Kelowna clear of rocks.[65] In Victoria, elderly, handicapped, and marginally employed men were given work as street cleaners.[66]

These employment opportunities, which were clearly a critical element of the survival strategies of many single old men in B.C., seem to have dried up by the end of the 1920s. The introduction of old age pensions in 1927 perhaps justified the elimination of this earlier form of assistance. Increased mechanization – the City of Victoria purchased a mechanical sweeper in 1926 and pensioned off its street sweepers – may have cut manual work on provincial roads as well. Or perhaps old men like the Vernon–Kelowna rock-picker were absorbed in the huge swamp of Depression relief recipients.

Michael Katz has labelled the inmates of nineteenth-century American workhouses the "casualties" of the emerging waged labour market.[67] I think this interpretation can also be applied to the aging labourers of British Columbia in the first half of the twentieth century. Resource capitalism provided employment for young fit men, but once they were older and no longer strong it had no place for them.

OLD WOMEN ALONE

Older women do not figure prominently in B.C.'s welfare records. In general, relief records speak to that which is absent, not that which is present. People who go to the state in need are those without anywhere else to turn. Deserted mothers and single old men were the most typical recipients of state assistance during the 1920s, the period most fully covered by the records of the provincial Indigent Fund. Few of the aged women whose lives are chronicled in welfare documents appear to have been as socially isolated or as economically vulnerable as their male cohorts or younger women on their own with children to support. Most daughters and sons who featured in the cases of old women did offer some assistance to their aged mothers. And when there was no kin to give support, neighbours and members of the local community often stepped in, providing employment, food, and shelter.

This pattern speaks both to gendered perceptions of old age and need and to the demography of old age in the province. Historians have noted that, because the female population has typically had an older age structure, when we talk of the elderly – both in the past and today – we are mostly referring to women.[68] In British Columbia, however, where men dominated the ranks of the province's elderly until 1960, the reverse was true. Old women were a smaller group and comparatively rare, especially in the isolated rural areas of the province.

The statistical analysis available indicates that old women in B.C. were likely to be widows. There were high rates of marriage for non-aboriginal women: in 1900, for example, approximately 80 per cent of white women in the province were either married or widowed.[69] Non-aboriginal women of this early period often married men who were considerably older than themselves.[70] By 1930 many of the young women who had married older men would be dealing with aging partners or living as aging women without partners.

Historically, at all stages of the life cycle most women were bound closely to the world of kin and home. Women's paid work was viewed as less important than male work and their roles in the family were

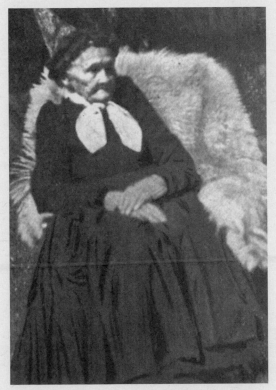

Mrs "Granny" Parker, an early resident at the Home
for Aged and Infirm Ladies, Victoria, no date. Taken
from an early history of the institution, Parker is
presented here as a worthy case for this philanthropic
establishment. (British Columbia Provincial Archives)

as wives, daughters, and mothers, not breadwinners. Life changes for
women, then, were linked to family, not work.[71] Their lives as elders
followed the pattern set in the middle years of their lives.

Since the lives of old women on their own are not as fully documented in the public record in B.C. as are the lives of single men, their
portrayal here is impressionistic rather than definitive. Nonetheless,
I think it is important to look at women when they were by themselves,
set apart from the kinship structures that so strongly defined the lives
of most women. A focus on aging women in this situation allows us
to isolate their options outside the bonds of family, to see clearly their
incredible vulnerability, and to consider how the larger community
took responsibility for them.

Single aged women held on tightly to what monetary assets they had
gained over their young and middle years. Katherine MacMillan wrote

to the provincial minister of Mines for help in 1923. Citing her historical significance as the first female prospector in her region, MacMillan said she had worked as a prospector in the Kootenays since 1891. Now she was over sixty years of age, unable to work because of illness, and was asking for financial assistance so that she might keep her claims going.[72]

But real estate, rather than mining claims, was the best economic asset for older women who were alone. Like the elderly elsewhere, women in B.C. used houses and land to generate ongoing income. I found several instances of subletting property as a form of income, just as Chris Gordon found for elderly men and women in London around 1930.[73] In 1917 a former nurse applying to enter the Home for Aged and Infirm Ladies told the home committee that the twenty-five-dollar monthly rent she received from a house in Winnipeg would cover her care.[74] In 1927 a prairie woman rented out her house in Manitoba for more than twice what she paid for rental accommodation on one of the Gulf Islands, and used her financial dividend to buy groceries and fuel.[75] An older single woman in Victoria two decades later was able to rent out her house for fifteen dollars each month and live in cheaper rental accommodation.[76] But these practices still required money for property taxes and were affected by shifting market conditions. A Victoria spinster thought her old age was economically secure with a life interest in a quarter section of land on the prairies, but by 1933 the Depression had eroded all income from this inheritance.[77]

B.C.'s resource-based economy, with large numbers of transient male labourers, meant that a large house was a valuable asset in a community where boarding accommodation was required. Mining communities in particular provided a good economic opportunity for boarding house operators. As Bettina Bradbury has illustrated, taking in boarders is a traditional female contribution to the family economy and is employed at different stages of the life cycle.[78] In old age, with the family home vacated by grown children, taking in boarders was a sensible economic strategy for women in B.C. A Slav widow without children and Canadian kin was able to keep boarders in her four-room Fernie home in the 1920s.[79] Another widow in the coal mining community of Wellington on Vancouver Island built and operated a profitable seventeen-room boarding house when the Pacific Coast Coal Mines were operating.[80] Both these women were without a male wage earner. Using property that they owned to generate an income meant that they could continue to live autonomously as they grew old.

There were no older working women with living spouses and few with children among the welfare records that I consulted, indicating that for many people it was not acceptable for a married woman to work for wages outside the home. Widows and spinsters, particularly immigrant women, were most likely to require income from paid work in old age, but formal waged labour was an unlikely option for them. Nationally, women over sixty-five were only a tiny proportion of the formal labour market: they never reached more than 7 per cent of female workers appearing in the census between 1921 and 1941.[81] Women of any age had few mainstream employment opportunities in B.C.'s resource communities,[82] so older women were doubly disadvantaged when they looked for paid work.

Instead, older women found informal waged work that mirrored female tasks performed at home: they took care of children, cleaned houses, did needlework, and cooked to maintain themselves. This kind of marginal domestic work may have been a strategy these women first adopted in their middle years. Mrs Bell, a widow residing at the Home for Aged and Infirm Ladies, left to take up a housekeeping position in May 1919.[83] An Okanagan woman worked variously during the 1920s as a housekeeper for a local priest, a baker, and a seamstress.[84] A woman in Midway did chores for people in the community.[85] The informal, local character of the work done by these women suggests that employment may have been offered to older women in need as a kind of ad hoc charitable measure.

Older women in urban communities, clearly examples of the "deserving" poor, could sometimes obtain charitable work. An elderly spinster in Victoria in 1933, one of the worst years of the Depression, found employment at the municipal Women's Work Room.[86] Spencers, a Victoria department store, also had a workroom where elderly women were employed. In 1943 an elderly woman was able to make nine dollars weekly there, but was let go when her health worsened.[87]

These stories have emphasized the initiative of old women in the fight to hold onto their independence, sometimes helped by sympathetic people in the local community. But in reality, elderly women whose lives had separated them from family were extremely vulnerable to poverty, ill health, and institutionalization; they were, as historian Stormi Stewart aptly puts it, in double jeopardy.[88] A provincial charge along with her aging husband since she was seventy, Elizabeth Todd was eighty years old when she entered the Home for Aged and Infirm Ladies in Victoria in 1920. She had been widowed less than two weeks and had no children.[89] In the case of older women like Todd who became widows, as Chudacoff and Hareven note, the critical event propelling them into an institution was not old age itself but the death of a male spouse.[90]

Welfare records contain cases of terrible destitution among elderly women without family. A neighbour in the interior of the province,

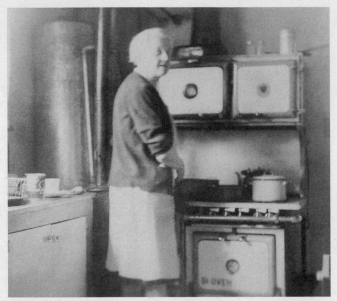

Dorthea (Dodo) McBride in the kitchen of Westminster House, ca
1943. Photographic images of old women in B.C. are hard to find,
reflecting the way in which women, and particularly aged working
women, are often hidden from history. This picture shows McBride
at work in the kitchen, doing the kind of home-centred labour that
characterized the working lives of elderly women. (City of New
Westminster photo collection)

reporting an elderly widow who "brought over a washstand and
traded it to Mrs T for some odd bits of clothing," was speaking of a
woman in desperate straits.[91] Similarly, an eighty-two-year-old Nelson
woman who sold her household effects in order that she could buy
groceries was clearly facing starvation.[92]

For all their economic vulnerability, however, older women on their
own rarely appear to have been as socially marginal as many of their
male counterparts. My evidence suggests that single older women on
B.C.'s economic margins did not move around like many of their
unmarried male cohorts, and were more integrated in their local community support systems. This was as much a reflection of paternalistic
social attitudes toward women as it was a testament to the transiency
of many men on their own.[93] In the eyes of the community a solitary
old woman was apparently *always* perceived as a person in need.
Notions of respectability may have not always been a major issue
when an elderly woman on her own was in distress. A case from Atlin
in 1920 indicates how community support for an old woman functioned

beyond the bounds of racial difference. The local government agent provided fuel and other kinds of assistance to an increasingly blind and deaf seventy-five-year-old black woman who was living in a small shack on the outskirts of town. Other members of the community also kept an eye on the woman, rescuing her when she set her cabin alight in mid-winter.[94]

Single aging women may have been a disadvantaged minority in B.C., but they were often resourceful and hard-working in their struggle to avoid institutionalization. Strategies for remaining independent included a careful use of assets obtained earlier in life and informal waged work. At the close of their lives, women performed a range of "female" tasks – work they might previously have done as wives and mothers – and cobbled together a livelihood. Old women who had no kin were more vulnerable than their male cohorts: an aged woman without waged work or property that she could barter into food and shelter was in an extremely precarious situation. It seems likely, however, that an elderly woman in this situation would be acknowledged as "deserving" and given assistance from people in the local community.

MARRIAGE AND FAMILY

Marriage and family were decisive in shaping the last decades of life. A home and a spouse were reasonable guarantees against institution-alization in a period of crisis. Couples were more likely to continue living independently in old age than were single men and women.[95] A 1948 survey of 1,000 social assistance cases in the Vancouver area found that 39 per cent of the married couples studied lived in their own home whereas only 4 per cent of single men and women were residing in an independent dwelling.[96] Grown children were another stabilizing factor. As historians of old age have found elsewhere, most daughters and sons were willing to take some responsibility for the care of their aged parents.[97]

The case of a husband and wife, both in their seventies, who lived in Cranbrook during the 1920s illustrates how a home and partner could provide financial and emotional stability in old age. The government agent who interviewed them noted their attachment to each other, the fact that they owned their own small house, and the husband's limited income from carpentry and cabinet making.[98] While not all marriages were companionable in old age, it is clear that marital assets accumulated in young and middle age provided financial stability when a couple grew old.

As with single men and women, property was a cornerstone of economic well-being for these aged people. A home that had been purchased outright, like the little cottage owned by the Cranbrook couple, was a solid guarantee of shelter, a roof over one's head in good and bad times. If an elderly person grew ill but was living in their own home with a spouse, the likelihood that they would be institutionalized was greatly diminished. The Todds, supported by the Indigent Fund from 1910 to 1920, were able to live independently during this period.[99]

Land could also be a productive resource. Older couples in B.C. used their land to supplement their limited incomes and to ensure a better diet than they would likely have had otherwise.[100] Into the 1930s and probably later, the wider suburbs of Vancouver and Victoria gave homeowners a cheap piece of land with room for livestock, fruit trees, and a garden. One popular location for the elderly of modest means was Maple Ridge, where "retirees lived in comfortable 'cottages,' each on an acre or more of land."[101]

Such activities were not, of course, limited to aged men and women who had marital partners. But the pattern of a settled, secure existence was more typical of married people than of those who were single. A British couple who had immigrated in 1888 spent their old age at Cobble Hill with a house, five acres of land, a couple of goats and hens, a good garden, and some productive fruit trees.[102] With all this they could produce their own milk, fruit, eggs, and vegetables. Careful management of the garden and storage in the mild climate of the Cowichan Valley could have garnered them vegetables for much of the year. Other elderly couples, like the Cooks at One Mile Creek near Princeton in the late 1920s, earned a small income from chickens and dairy products.[103]

Marriage anchored old men more firmly in a specific locale, making them respectable in the eyes of the community and apparently eligible for a different kind of assistance than their single counterparts.[104] There are few instances of married men finding work on provincial roads, employment that would likely have taken them away from their homes during the summer months. In 1914, when his general store closed, Stephen Spender was appointed janitor at the local courthouse with a monthly salary of twenty-five dollars. At seventy-six Spender could not hope to find other employment, and the fact that he and his wife had been pioneer settlers in the valley meant that they were "deserving" recipients for such aid.[105] The respectability of marriage may also have made elderly couples more attractive to people who wanted live-in help, like the proprietor of an Okanagan hotel who employed Caroline and Charles Wilder to care for the establishment during the winter. The Wilders were given no monetary compensation for their work, but had milk, butter, eggs, and fuel, and a free place to live.[106]

Grown offspring often gave critical support to aged parents. With financial support and practical assistance from their children, an elderly couple could continue to live independently. A Nanaimo couple interviewed in 1925 by the local constable had the stability of their own house and five acres of land. But because the husband had been unable to work for four years, they depended on fifteen dollars sent monthly by each of their five sons.[107] In a time of crisis, family assistance could be pivotal. When Alice and Jack Kendal's Vancouver home was destroyed by fire, one son gave them a house to live in and another bought them furniture and food.[108] For the Kendals, aged sixty-five and seventy-six, this support ensured their ongoing autonomy.

These cases from Nanaimo and Vancouver show strong family commitment to aged parents, but other situations were more complex. Grown sons and daughters did not automatically accept responsibility for their elders. Assistance was calculated on what family resources were available and the perceived need of the elderly person in question. Some offspring held back from giving help as long as their parent was capable of earning money, like the Nanaimo man whose mother worked as a nurse and then came to live in a cabin owned by her son.[109] An Alberni woman responded sharply to the government agent who questioned her about her parents' financial position in 1923: with two sisters and a brother she was not solely responsible for her parents, the elderly couple had never asked her for help, nor was she able to give assistance. Furthermore, while she was "always willing to do my share when the time comes ... at the present moment I do not think it is as bad as you state."[110] As Chudacoff and Hareven have noted, children were often trying to establish themselves with a home and a family at the same time that their elderly parents needed help holding onto their own autonomy. Conflicting sets of intergenerational needs could easily result in discord between older parents and middle-aged children.[111]

Historians have employed the family economy model to explain how intergenerational families have functioned in the past.[112] This construct is useful for understanding the ways in which B.C. families strategized to give support to aged parents and, at the same time, ensure that the family as a whole benefited from the situation. Property could form the basis of negotiation and assistance, as it did in 1927 in the case of a son who was buying his parents' fruit farm by paying their rent and giving them thirty dollars each month to live on.[113] Inheritances were sometimes arranged to safeguard the interests of both the parent and the child who would eventually inherit, like the elderly woman in the northern region of the province who had been left the family ranch jointly with her son. Living only fifty yards away from her son's house, and connected to the main dwelling by telephone, this woman had the dual security of family support and an established place to live.[114]

Some extended families worked out complex systems of intergenerational exchange. One East Vancouver household of the 1940s and

1950s included a maternal grandmother who lived on the top floor and a paternal grandfather who lived in the basement. The grandmother brought in wages from her job at the Hotel Vancouver and did housekeeping, cooking, and childcare. The grandfather, who had built the house during the Second World War, used his carpentry skills to construct homes nearby for his brother and his son. In exchange for their contributions, the older man and woman were given a place to live, meals, and emotional support.[115]

Some families exchanged services for money. During the Second World War a couple in Chase were paid twenty-five dollars to care for their granddaughter while her mother worked as a nurse and her father served overseas.[116] Historians argue that old women like the grandmother in Chase were welcomed into the family home because they could make a valuable contribution by helping with housework and childcare – tasks that old men were unable or unwilling to undertake.[117] The case of Mary Black illuminates the ways in which an older woman could provide essential services within the home. Black, a widow, came out to B.C. during the First World War to live with her married daughter while the daughter's husband was overseas. When the daughter died Black continued to keep house for the widowed husband and her grandchild until the father married again.[118]

Another model of care for elderly parents is help given in exchange for past services rendered. This "welfare" model of assistance is based on the affectionate ties and obligations due to an aging and vulnerable parent rather than a reciprocal relationship. Michael Anderson argues that families based what they could give on the resources they had at their disposal.[119] Grown offspring in B.C. gave both personal care and financial assistance to their aged parents, but set boundaries to their generosity as well. Typically, a crisis would lead to a reassessment of the care relationship, perhaps rendering a long-standing arrangement unworkable. Two daughters, for example, provided shelter, food, and clothing for their seventy-year-old father from 1922 until he grew ill in 1926. At that point they told the local police constable that they were willing to pay for the operation that their father needed, but could not continue to give ongoing support.[120] Similarly, Alfred Stacey, who entered the Old Men's Home just before Christmas in 1937, had lived with his married daughter for two years. Now his daughter was ill herself and no longer able to care for him.[121]

Family support took a number of forms, showing that families employed diverse strategies to accommodate the needs of aged kin. Some older people lived with married children, like the seventy-eight-year-old Fernie woman who found a clean and comfortable home with her married daughter in 1927.[122] Another family investigated in the same year had worked collectively to care for their aging mother, taking turns to give her a home, as none were able to keep her full-time.[123] Three unmarried sons made their base at their mother's farm near Hazelton in northern British Columbia, returning home between labouring jobs in the local area. Their father having died one year previously, the sons informed the investigating police constable that they had always supported their mother and would continue to do so.[124]

As these cases suggest, the B.C. data supports the common historical argument that female relatives were perceived as more needy in old age and were more easily accommodated within the family than were elderly men.[125] The work of caring that they had done as mothers was now due to be repaid. The Home for Aged and Infirm Ladies' minute books give us glimpses of the centrality of family in the care of older female kin. A son in Revelstoke applied for his mother to enter the institution in July 1901. She stayed only a month before leaving to reside with her daughter.[126] The daughter of Mrs Scolton expressed her surprise when her mother entered the Home in 1916, telling the committee that she had expected to maintain her mother in old age.[127]

Family affection and love are particularly evident in the sacrifices daughters made for their mothers. Some daughters gave money and lodging to their mothers. Others took on the difficult task of making a long-term commitment to care for a mother in frail health, a pattern that echoes data found by Peter Townsend in his 1957 British study of old people and families.[128] The case of Evelyn Thornburn and her daughter demonstrates the range of care and support that daughters gave to their mothers. Thornburn, a Scot, immigrated to Canada to join her daughters in Fernie after her husband died. At that point she became totally dependent on one daughter, having no bank account, no personal property, and no source of income. In 1927, when Thornburn was seventy-six and very frail, the local member of the Legislative Assembly wrote to ask for provincial aid, stating that "the daughter has broken her health in trying to help her mother as well as attend to her family and it is impossible for her to continue doing so."[129]

The case of Nancy Miller also illustrates the role daughters took in caring for their mothers and shows how sisters worked together to find appropriate situations. In 1945 Miller's daughter Emily Boutroy asked if her mother could enter the Provincial Infirmary. Miller, who had lived with the Boutroy family for more than fourteen years, had been ill over the winter and was no longer able to recognize her relatives. The family hoped that she would go to the Provincial Infirmary at Marpole, where another daughter was a nurse and would be able to care for her mother.[130] It is likely that both Miller and Thornburn had been contributory members of their daughters' families until ill health forced them into a welfare relationship.

While these stories show families readily giving care and affection to their aged parents, the family home could also become a contested space, with frustrated and unhappy elders in conflict with younger kin. As Michael Anderson has noted, relationships that were not perceived as reciprocal were liable to create stress within the family unit.[131] I envision that as Miller and Thornburn grew more frail and needy, the stress on their daughters' families grew substantially. Indeed, the 1927 missive from the local MLA depicts Thornburn's beleaguered daughter struggling in her multiple roles as nurse, daughter, mother, wife, and housekeeper.

Family friction also emerged over questions of control and domestic space, important issues for old women used to having their own homes and kitchens.[132] Not all women were willing to give up their house or were keen to share space with married offspring and their families. A Vancouver police corporal who was trying to find a home for an aging woman in 1926 found that "it is hopeless to ask the mother to live with either of her daughters-in-law as they cannot agree."[133] The following year a frustrated man in Port Alice reported that his mother refused to reside with his wife and him and insisted instead on living in an old shack.[134] This last story shows how offspring and dependent parents could have very different agendas: for the mother, the essential issue was autonomy, while her son had concerns about respectability and his mother's well-being.

An analysis of the importance of family in old age shows the impact of steps taken midway through life upon the final stage of the life cycle. Clearly, marriage and family paid off decisive dividends in old age. Although there were no certainties at the close of life, the real and personal assets of a home, a spouse, and offspring tended to make old age more settled and financially secure, and elderly people less vulnerable to institutionalization.

COMMUNITY SUPPORT IN OLD AGE

Elderly men and women also turned to members of their local community for help. Suzanne Morton found little evidence of community support for the needy in working-class Halifax during the 1920s,[135] but I, like James Snell, was struck by the role played by neighbours, government agents, and provincial policemen in assisting the aged, particularly in B.C.'s rural communities.[136] "Community" is an elusive term, but my evidence suggests that social systems that benefited the aged worked differently in rural and urban settings.[137] Older residents were known as individuals in smaller towns and rural locales. They were acknowledged as pioneer citizens with the right to assistance in old age, and local aid was often crafted to suit individual needs. Community responsibility for elders worked differently in larger urban centres, where older women and men were both less visible and more likely to be cared for by members of their own ethnic or social group.

In smaller, rural settlements regular faces and characters were firmly implanted in the public mind. Old people were remembered and their state of health and absence noted. In 1924 the government agent in Lumby wrote to the superintendent of the Provincial Home to inquire as to the whereabouts of Percy Gareau: friends and neighbours of the former Lumby resident had not heard from him for some time and were anxious for news.[138] Community attention to the elderly echoed down through the twentieth century. Notification of the death of Fred Newton in 1961, a former blacksmith and old-timer on Mayne Island who had gone to live in the Provincial Home for Aged Men, was tacked up on the post office noticeboard for all to see.[139]

An important feature of this kind of local memory was a sense of responsibility toward residents who had been early pioneers and were now old, sick, or poor. Petitions to the provincial secretary for funds often included an acknowledgment of the pioneering role played by the now aged settler. After Samuel Sunderland died in 1926, for example, the local government agent requested assistance for his widow, stating that "Mr and Mrs S came into the ... Valley in 1873, being amongst the early settlers in this district, and have had to undergo the many hardships attendant to pioneering in this upper country. Mrs S is entitled to any consideration which could, properly, in order and in your good judgement be extended to her."[140] This kind of request for assistance linked ordinary elderly British Columbians to the heroic work of nation-building on the edge of a new land.

This "welfare" support for people who had become elders in a tight-knit locality was similar to children repaying aged parents for rearing them. Family responsibility, with kin often far away from B.C., was transposed onto the local community. In smaller settlements communal work done by older people when they were young and fit was remembered and seen as worthy of compensation. A resident of the Invermere Valley, writing to the local member of the Legislative Assembly on behalf of a widowed neighbour, referred to debts owed by "the many residents of this Valley who were helped by her in days gone by."[141]

Without local charitable groups to do the work of caring for the aged, rural people came together to seek funds for impoverished elderly people whom they considered worthy of assistance. In 1923 three Keremeos residents asked the attorney general to help a seventy-three-year-old local man who had worked in the province for twenty-three years but was no longer able to support himself.[142] This kind of collective undertaking appears to have been relatively common in rural areas and entirely the work of men.

Individual character, as measured by the local community, could be a critical determinant in this process. Characteristics like a willingness to work hard and a drive for independence, both part of the classic frontier ethos, were seen as positive attributes.[143] A 1927 petition co-authored by Salmon Arm's justice of the peace and a fellow resident on behalf of a seventy-six-year-old widow highlighted these personal qualities: "She is a very independent old dame, there are not many like her, neither are there many in her condition who would have struggled along as she has done."[144]

Rural neighbours, usually women, stepped in to provide valuable practical assistance for the aged and infirm.[145] As James Snell notes, community assistance was available to cover a short-term crisis. If dependence continued and there was no help from family, then community members would look to the state for help.[146] When Robert Marland became ill, the bachelor farmer was nursed at home by Mrs Hovis, a neighbour. Although Mrs Hovis believed that her friend "should make up his mind to go to a home, where he would be well cared for and get the sort of nourishment an old man requires to keep strength up," her care meant that he did not have to enter an institution. Marland died before institutionalization became inevitable, but the local doctor, hospital administrators, and the provincial police constable were involved in discussions about transferring the old man to the Provincial Home.[147]

Outside the city, with its municipal relief systems and philanthropic enterprises, individual women took on the practical work of urban charities. Women cooked meals, cleaned, and did laundry for their elderly bachelor neighbours.[148] Helen Brown, the wife of a contractor in Fort Steele, wrote to her bachelor neighbour at the Provincial Home in 1923 to say she would provide him with meals if he wanted to come home and live in his cabin nearby. Just let her know in good time, Brown warned her friend, so she could have the "shack" all tidy for his arrival.[149]

In isolated places watch was kept on the aged through an informal network of neighbours, friends, government agents, and provincial police constables. This kind of care does not seem to have excluded transients, suggesting a more malleable notion of community than one might expect in a small settlement. In 1927 the local provincial police constable in Quesnel wrote that an elderly prospector was overdue for a visit to town and known to be short of food.[150] His report, like many others, indicates that information was passed on by another party, perhaps a friend or acquaintance of the elderly man. Provincial police were vigilant in their care of old men and women, even giving practical assistance with gathering fuel and clearing snow.[151] Elderly people and their neighbours sometimes worked out mutually advantageous schemes, like the old woman at Secret Cove outside Vancouver who allowed local fishers to use her bay as anchorage in exchange for wood, fish, and meat.[152] Again, such reciprocal agreements between neighbours mirrored arrangements made among kin.

The experience of elderly men and women on the margins was different in urban settings. As Graeme Wynn has noted, in the urban milieu social systems were organized around "insiders" and "outsiders."[153] In B.C.'s towns and cities, "community" was defined by neighbourhood, place of work, leisure pursuits, and church attendance. Moreover, as R.A.J. McDonald makes clear in the case of Vancouver, a strong racist creed divided the urban setting into ethnic enclaves. This understanding of urban communities as a set of "local social systems" makes sense of the life stories I discovered.[154] Older people looked to what they defined as their particular community for identification and support. The elderly with a strong place within an urban community could count on assistance; socially marginal people had less recourse to help.

The case of a blind Greek bachelor in Victoria is a good illustration of how ethnic bonds worked. The seventy-five-year-old man had been living with another Greek man in a waterfront shack. His friend was now in hospital, but the city social worker found that "various Greek men have been going down to his shack with food, etc."[155] Community, here defined by male ethnic bonds rather than by neighbourhood or class, fostered a strong sense of responsibility to an aging compatriot in need.

I found little information about informal support for the aged in other ethnic communities in B.C., but it is reasonable to assume that elderly Italians, Chinese, and East Indians, less integrated into Anglo-Saxon British Columbia than Scandinavian immigrants, would turn to their compatriots when they needed help. What published secondary sources do suggest, however, is that settled, "mature" immigrant communities with intergenerational families were sometimes uncomfortable with older bachelors, men they often themselves perceived as rough and unrespectable. Robert Harney tells us that "[w]hile most Italian communities in North America have a few old unmarried 'uncles' and *cafoni* who are the fossils of that earlier abnormal life style, Italian culture has not been tolerant of bachelorhood."[156] As the members of male ethnic communities died off, critical networks of support for single old men may have disappeared.

Respectable couples, widows, and spinsters living lives of quiet poverty were attractive to middle-class philanthropists. A private Victoria charity run by a small group of women paid for three women at the Home for Aged and Infirm Ladies and another at Miss Martin's boarding house in the 1920s. All of the women had been residents of the city for at least forty years.[157] The Ladies' Benevolent Society in Fernie cared for an elderly local couple in the same period.[158]

Boarding houses, where many urban elderly on minimal incomes lived, were another form of support demarcated on class and gender lines. Miss Martin, who kept women boarders in the genteel area near the Anglican cathedral during the 1930s, gave room, board, and some nursing care to elderly spinsters.[159] The Clifton Rooms and the Salvation Army Hostel were in a different part of Victoria and housed older working men, but the proprietors of these boarding houses, too, kept an eye on the well-being of their elderly clients. In February 1937, for example, five proprietors of Vancouver boarding houses reported that they had pensioners who required medical attention.[160]

Despite the many instances of community working *for* old people, however, ageism is a common theme in historical work on societal attitudes and practices toward aged people. Arlene Tigar McLaren's oral history of neighbourhood life in East Vancouver tells of an elderly woman labeled "the Witch" by local children. The fact that the woman was old, lived in a dilapidated farmhouse, and had no kinship links within the neighbourhood set her apart from the local community.[161] Suzanne Morton, focusing on the divide between generations in her writing on 1920s working-class Halifax, gives a much more negative view of community attitudes toward elderly people.[162]

An examination of police and judicial records and further oral histories of community life in B.C. might reveal a more nuanced picture than the one I have presented here. Nonetheless, it is clear that community often worked in favour of old people, usually through the agency of women. Community awareness of the plight of the impoverished elderly was common in both rural and urban settings, but assistance worked rather differently in each case. Long-time residents in rural settlements could trade their personal investment in the local community for care and support in old age. In the urban locale assistance for the infirm and indigent aged was more structured, and communities of support were more narrowly defined around neighbourhood, class, and ethnicity.

STATE SUPPORT FOR THE AGED

Elderly women and men also turned to the state for help. The options available to them, and the philosophical basis for state assistance, shifted considerably over the period covered by this book. The regimented, moralistic character of early state care was moderated by a paternalistic concern and a measure of respect for the aged. Old age pensions, introduced in 1927, marked the first application of modern welfare state principles to elderly British Columbians. The pension, undoubtedly a boon to the aged poor, drew old people into the net of the corporate welfare state.

Elderly men and women living independently in unorganized areas of the province before 1927 could petition for money from the provincial Indigent Fund, a system of outdoor poor relief that was later replaced by the old age pension. Established in 1880 and administered by the deputy provincial secretary, the fund gave money to those who were unable to provide for themselves; the elderly were a primary beneficiary of the fund. Assistance was given to old people who did not wish to enter a public institution and to those who had a home in which to live but no income.[163] During the 1920s, the period best documented, there appears to have been a fairly liberal distribution of the fund: money was given to elderly indigents from a range of ethnic groups, and assistance was handled in a relatively sensitive manner.

The Indigent Fund is a good illustration of pre-welfare state paternalism and poor law principles. Administrators of the fund did not question the legitimacy of poverty; the old were often poor after all. Ostensibly, recipients were to be destitute individuals whose moral qualities made them worthy of aid, and state assistance was to be as unattractive as possible to discourage dependency.[164] That the fund was used to help old people with property but no money, however, illustrates the flexibility and benevolence that were essential characteristics of this early welfare system.

Yet the ethos of the Poor Law was also a strong characteristic of the way in which the fund was administered. Communication between government agents, police constables, and the deputy provincial secretary frequently reverted to the discourse of the Poor Law. They would note that the man in question was in ill health and unable to work, but also comment on his moral character. Mention might be made of the "exemplary habits" of an applicant, or (in the case of one man) that he was "very seldom seen around the Beer Parlour."[165] Aid was sometimes controlled by a local merchant for, as one government agent commented in a 1927 case of an old man, "I would not trust him with a nickel, for as soon as he gets his hands on money he develops an unquenchable thirst for anything with a kick."[166]

David Roberts has noted the importance of personal relationships, hierarchies of power, and "smallness" in paternalist systems.[167] Viewed in this manner, the individualized and local nature of early welfare iniatives like the Indigent Fund becomes apparent. Government agents, friends, members of the community, and local charity associations made requests for assistance from the Indigent Fund. Their personal knowledge of the old man or woman in need was critical to the legitimacy of the claim. To further establish the credentials of the needy, those inquiring often noted that the old person in question was one of the region's early prospectors or settlers. When the government agent in Merritt wrote in 1926 on behalf of two elderly settlers he stated that they were among the first non-aboriginals to arrive in the valley and "had to undergo the many hardships attendant to pioneering in this upper country."[168] This kind of local advocacy also meant that the community sat in judgment of who needed and who deserved help. Government agents and police constables, in particular, were in the position of being able to use the fund in a highly personal fashion, obtaining aid or blocking access as they saw fit.

Applications were judged and awards made on an individual basis, another facet of paternalism. Racial origin was apparently not a decisive factor in determining if aid would be given: I found no instances of aboriginal people receiving funds, for they would have been under the jurisdiction of the federal Department of Indian Affairs, but otherwise there were cases from across the ethnic spectrum. In 1925, for example, the government agent in Smithers investigated the case, mentioned earlier, of the penniless Chinese miner who was living with First Nations people at Fort Babine. The sum of ten dollars a month was allocated to the Babine Hudson's Bay store to provide the necessary provisions for the man.[169] Two years later, because he was not a British subject, the elderly Chinese miner would have been denied assistance under the new old age pensions program, but the more flexible system in 1925 ensured him a means of survival.

The provincial policy of paying neighbours and relatives for the care of the elderly was a similar mixture of benevolence and government budgeting. Administrators appreciated that home and community were important to old people and were also aware that limited monthly payments to caregivers were a smaller drain on the state than institutionalization. In this earlier stage of state development, when personalized systems prevailed, women were paid to be agents of the state for the elderly in the community. In 1919 the deputy provincial secretary responded to a request from a sixty-five-year-old woman living south of Nanaimo. The woman's husband had declared that he was unable to give his ailing wife a home, and the Nanaimo hospital was no longer willing to accommodate her. The provincial secretary's office suggested that her friends be offered a small allowance in exchange for taking the woman into their home.[170]

Another way in which the Indigent Fund worked for older people was the attitude of administrators toward property. Some recipients owned small plots of land but were unable to support themselves.[171] Here again, the state generally found it cheaper to give a minimal monthly cash payment than pay for institutional accommodation.[172] Thus the Jameses of Cobble Hill on Vancouver Island, brought to the attention of the provincial secretary in 1924, were a good investment for the state. With a productive garden, chickens, and goats, the British couple only needed some small financial aid to remain independent.[173]

As the above cases suggest, the administrative flexibility of the fund allowed for prompt responses that were fashioned to meet the particular circumstances of B.C.'s rural elderly poor. Because applications were judged and rates set on an individual basis, aid could be given quickly and appropriately. In August 1922, for example, the government agent in Smithers reported that a local man, sixty-four years old, had been "stricken with paralysis" and was living in a rooming house on his last few dollars. The province agreed to cover the man's rent and pay a local restaurant to provide his meals.[174] In 1925 a seventy-six-year-old German man living in a shack near Fauquier was allocated seven dollars per month to spend at Needles Stores during the winter season. Help was not needed during the warm summer months, when the man could find work and provide for himself.[175]

In Victoria and Vancouver the elderly with limited resources could also turn to civic relief agencies for help. Organized municipal assistance for Vancouver's sick and destitute was established in 1888 and administered by the medical health officer until 1895, when the work was taken over by the Friendly Help Society. The society changed its name to Associated Charities of Vancouver in 1909. Victoria's Friendly Help Association was active from the late nineteenth century, and a sister association was established in the neighbouring municipality of Esquimalt in 1912. Saanich, another municipality that borders Victoria, had an active Friendly Help Association during the Depression years.[176] These groups operated as quasi-state organizations, relying on municipal governments for regular funding but operating independently with support from local individuals and businesses.[177] Like Friendly Help Associations elsewhere in the country, these agencies provided outdoor relief to the indigent elderly in the form of money, food, clothing, household items, and casual employment.

This co-operation between the state and the voluntary sector evolved differently in Vancouver and Victoria. In both cases, the scheme initially allowed the municipality to back away from giving charity directly to the indigent aged, an activity that many municipal politicians assumed would attract the sick and destitute to their cities. This was what British historian Geoffrey Finlayson would call co-operation based on negative principles, the desire to save money and discourage dependency.[178] While the continued use of state funds to shore up the voluntary sector, a particular characteristic of early urban welfare systems in western Canada, was successful in Victoria and its neighbouring municipalities, it was not viable in the larger community of Vancouver.[179] By 1915 Associated Charities had become part of Vancouver's Social Service Department.

Like other people who lived outside the social and moral sphere of the white, middle-class family, the aged indigent was often regarded as socially problematic in the urban milieu of Vancouver. A 1909 Vancouver news article, for example, decried the fact that old male indigents spent their days on the streets begging drinks in saloons, getting drunk, and selling alcohol to aboriginal people.[180] State assistance, therefore, worked as both carrot and stick to police the behaviour of aging people who lived on the margins of urban society. In the early twentieth century, at any rate, an elderly applicant would not necessarily find it easy to obtain assistance in Vancouver. Older people were expected to support themselves or look to their families for help. If relatives could be found elsewhere then the elderly applicant would be relocated out of Vancouver's municipal jurisdiction. In the late 1930s civic administrators told relief applicants over sixty years of age that the only help they would receive was admission to the unpopular municipal Old People's Home.[181]

In spite of the harsh character of its civic relief system, Vancouver attracted aged transients with limited financial resources because the city was familiar and offered social services that an elderly worker from the hinterland might require. During the Second World War Phyllis Knight met up with "Pat," a friend from her youth in the interior of the province, and found that he was now resident in Vancouver and living in a "run-down row cabin" that she called "The Black Hole of Calcutta."[182] The fact that Pat was able to obtain relief, however miserly, was one factor in his move to the city. The presence of the Salvation Army's Metropole Hostel, the Vancouver City Rescue Mission, and the Central City Mission, all supported by municipal funds, meant that Pat had a place to go if he fell on hard times.[183]

There is no evidence from Victoria to suggest similar attitudes toward the indigent elderly, perhaps a reflection of the smaller numbers of transients that made it across the Strait of Georgia. Old men and women deemed worthy of assistance were given help. In 1927, for example, Victoria's Friendly Help Association gave assistance to an old man who had come to Canada in 1879 with the Hudson's Bay Company.[184] Support might be temporary, as in the case of the Hudson's Bay man, or long term. Another impoverished Victoria resident, a sixty-eight-year-old man, was supported by the Friendly Help Society for a number of years before his case was taken over by civic relief officials in 1932.[185]

The introduction of old age pensions in B.C. in 1927 drew both urban and rural elders into a provincial system of assistance for the aged. British Columbia was the first province in Canada to participate in the federal program, introduced by Prime Minister Mackenzie King and his Liberal government under pressure from the two Labour members of Parliament, J.S. Woodsworth and A.A. Heaps. The new Old Age Pensions Act gave eligible old people a set monthly sum of twenty dollars. B.C. applicants were subjected to a means test by the Workmen's Compensation Board, but it appears that western pensions administrators were less strict than in Ontario and the Maritime provinces. Recipients had to be British subjects over the age of seventy who had lived in Canada for twenty years and in B.C. for five.[186]

The provincial pensions program brought together the old and the new in its approach toward state assistance to the aged. The systematic way in which applicants were selected, the dominance of a central bureaucracy, and the use of standard forms and specific procedures heralded the emergence of the corporate state in B.C.[187] Pension applicants were treated as individuals only in so much as they satisfied the criteria for assistance. Aid was no longer tailored to meet specific needs based on an individual's personal health and capability but was now linked to a specific numeric quantity imposed by the state. In seeking systematically to create a retired class of people within the larger populace, the new program meant that the state had engaged in structuring an age-stratified society.

The more problematic elements of the plan show that the Poor Law had not been entirely vanquished. Successful applicants were re-investigated every six months. The calculation of a monthly pension of twenty dollars with a limited amount of additional income permitted was based on the belief, held by government administrators but nowhere verified by research, that the elderly required only one dollar per day on which to live. This was not the case. So, even from the start, the old age pension was inadequate for the purpose it was designed for, reflecting the Poor Law notion that assistance should be as meagre as possible to discourage reliance on the state. While the value of the pension increased during the Depression, the 1940s were very hard times for those struggling to survive solely on a state pension.[188] The strict residency and citizenship requirements excluded elderly men and women who could not obtain the necessary papers and those who had come to Canada as immigrants from Europe and Asia and never become naturalized British subjects. Other aging people in poor health with limited incomes were not old enough to qualify.

State paternalism, another facet of the Poor Law, did not disappear with the advent of the old age pensions plan. Some theorists maintain that paternalism is incompatible with the welfare state, but the 1943 transformation of the provincial pension department from an accountancy function to a social service administration illustrates how older elements of paternalism found a new, professional expression within the corporate welfare state. Responsibility for pensions was taken away from the Workmen's Compensation Board, and a new board was created with a social service division to deal with pension applications and housing and health problems. With a detailed application form giving information about a variety of aspects of the pensioner's life, those implementing the new policy maintained that "the applicant could be seen as a human being, rather than a number."[189]

Over time, the personal relationship and the hierarchy of power that are characteristic of paternalism re-emerged most fully within the relationship between the elderly client and his or her social worker. Amy Edwards, the first supervisor of the new Social Service Department of the Provincial Pensions Department, argued that social workers should have wide-ranging involvement in the lives of their aged clients.[190] The elderly indigents were perceived as belonging to an earlier and simpler pioneer era and therefore as too "unworldly" to cope with modern society. In an increasingly competitive world, social workers maintained, the old age pensioner needed protection and guidance.[191] It was suggested that even the complex regulations governing assistance or pension application forms might overwhelm a person who had spent his or her life in an oral culture.[192] The bureaucrat and the social worker, connected with the urban milieu of the corporate state and the university, were ideal intermediaries between the solitary pioneer and the mid-twentieth-century community. Mrs Phillipa Reid, who metamorphosed from clerk to social worker at the main pension office in Vancouver, was noteworthy for her ability to work with elderly clients in this fashion.[193]

For those who were able to satisfy the application criteria, the monthly old age pension payments became a cornerstone of economic well-being and independent living.[194] Pensions were tremendously popular with the elderly because, although they were means tested, they appear to have been given directly to the recipient without moral judgment.[195] Recipients could therefore interpret the pension as a right rather than a form of charity or the hated Poor Law. Interviewing a ninety-year-old Scottish man at the time that pensions were introduced, a government agent reported that the man "does not want what he calls, Charity, but has no objections to the old age pension."[196] Provincial government reports of the period refer to the "growing pension-consciousness of the public," which was one reason for increased pension expenditures.[197]

What was more important for the new pensioners, however, was the fact that a regular monthly pension cheque provided a firm financial base for continued independence. Scholars in the field of aging and social policy argue that institutionalization is unnecessary in many cases if adequate food and shelter are provided.[198] Historians have considered the role played by old age pensions in reducing the numbers of healthy aged in institutions. Old age pensions were introduced in Britain in 1908: by 1912 the number of elderly men and women living in Poor Law facilities had fallen by 20 per cent.[199] Kenneth Bryden and Veronica Strong-Boag have each suggested that a similar pattern occurred in Canada, which the B.C. data confirm.[200] While good health and the ability to gain a small additional income remained critical, the old age pension often allowed elderly men or women to continue living in their own home, a hotel, or a rooming house.

Although Canadian historians have noted harsh attitudes toward pension recipients, by the 1940s a liberal approach had apparently been adopted in British Columbia.[201] During the decade state payments to the elderly gradually increased. In 1942 B.C. began paying pensioners an additional allowance of five dollars per month. In 1945 assistance was extended to people between the ages of sixty-five and sixty-nine who had limited financial resources, and free medical care was provided for all B.C. residents who received either old age assistance or an old age pension. Two years later the citizenship and residency requirements for old age pensions were widened. In 1951 the federal government scrapped the old age pension plan and brought in the Old Age Security Program and the Old Age Assistance Scheme. The first program was universal in scope, giving all people who had reached the age of seventy a pension, while the second allowed those between sixty-five and sixty-nine to apply for means-tested support. Thus, while elderly British Columbians edged closer to the universal welfare state, those approaching their seventies still had to contend with a legacy of the Poor Law.[202]

It is clear that the introduction of old age pensions was of great importance to elderly people. Over time there was a subtle but significant reordering of the life cycle of the vulnerable aged: impoverished old age no longer meant that institutionalization was likely. Theorists of old age and the welfare state like Peter Townsend and Chris Phillipson would have us believe that the pensions system created a structured dependency that robs the elderly of choice and freedom and sets them apart from the rest of society.[203] While, as stated in the introduction, I can appreciate the philosophical dimensions of this argument, it fails entirely to take into account the very difficult lives of elderly people without money or family in the pre-pension era. A pension allowed Matthew Barker to stay in his beloved cabin near Vernon in 1949.[204] A pension would have given Robert Marland of Saltspring Island the same luxury in 1919. The kindness of neighbours and money from the Indigent Fund allowed Marland to live out his life in his own home, but surely at some cost to his sense of personal dignity.[205] And over time, as Snell has pointed out, pensions would serve as a tool of politicalization among Canada's aged.

A number of factors shaped old age in B.C. and determined the like-lihood of an elderly person entering an institution in the final stage of life. Gender, marital status, the presence of children, health, and class – all of these were key variables in the way in which elderly men and women strategized to remain independent. Old people pieced together fragments of employment, charity, and relief work. Good health was always pivotal.

I found a distinct population of aging, single, labouring men in B.C. Some of these old men made seasonal or permanent migrations from hinterland to metropolis. There, they lived in boarding houses or cabins in areas of town they had frequented as young working men. Others chose to remain in remote settlements, making their homes in rough shacks and trapping and fishing. The extreme vulnerability of these men illuminates the harsh nature of resource capitalism in B.C.: old workers were simply cast off to form an underclass in the larger community. The situation of women in old age was quite different, for here the measure of vulnerability in old age was determined by the strength of the family system rather than the ability to work.

Overall, the presence of supportive family seems to have been the most important variable. Families provided critical help to aged kin in times of crisis and gave ongoing financial or practical assistance. But local communities also took on these roles, nurturing aged pioneers who they believed had won the right to an independent old age. Elderly men and women without ties to family or community were therefore particularly vulnerable to institutionalization.

Some scholars argue that social programs like old age pensions foster dependency and social isolation among the elderly. However, it is evident that monthly pension cheques gave many aged British Columbians a better bid for independence in the last phase of their lives. The growth of state assistance to the elderly outside the old age home was arguably the most significant change that took place in the lives of old people living in the community during the period from the 1890s to the 1950s. Yet we should set pensions on the historic continuum of state assistance, perhaps neither as immediately useful to the impoverished aged as the Indigent Fund nor as value-free as our own experience with universal pensions might have us believe.

2 Homes for Pioneers and Homes for Senior Citizens: Institutional Development

Institutions are curious, chameleon-like creatures, taking on new roles unthought of when the cornerstones were first laid, or emerging from obscurity as need arises. They can be a symbol of public pride one decade, the focus of incensed newspaper editorials the next, or ignored by all but a handful of government inspectors for their entire existence. The history of old age homes in British Columbia underscores the fact that the old age home, like most other institutions, is an evolving narrative, a story with a shifting plot.[1] Moreover, the elderly also found shelter in other institutional settings – the general hospital, the boarding house, and the private hospital. Miss Jane Marple, Agatha Christie's venerable spinster, once said, "if you are looking at one thing, you can't be looking at another."[2] Like the canny pensioner from St Mary's Mead, the historian of old age must turn detective and look for the aged in institutions that were not labelled "old age homes."

Old age homes have always been physical manifestations of social and cultural attitudes toward the last phase of life.[3] Late nineteenth- and early twentieth-century public institutions built for the elderly in B.C. appeared no different from the outside than other state residential facilities of the period: society did not yet perceive the elderly as distinct from the rest of the populace, so their accommodation was not designed with them in mind. In addition to purpose-built facilities, old age homes were also created out of "borrowed" buildings, existing structures marginally altered for their new purpose.

The number of borrowed institutions that became old age homes speaks to the low status of the aged. Over the inter-war years, as old age pensions allowed healthy people to continue living independently, both borrowed and created old age homes remade spaces within their walls for increasing numbers of infirm residents. It was not until high noon of the twentieth century, when old age emerged as a specific stage in the life cycle and one worthy of professional interest, that a distinct style of architecture for the old age home took shape.[4]

The first public and charitable facilities for aged British Columbians were built at the close of the nineteenth century, the focus of civic pride and a reflection of the belief that elderly pioneers had earned the right to die in some comfort. In this same period the new province was constructing other state institutions, like jails, hospitals, and insane asylums, visible symbols of the emerging social control state, and B.C.'s early old age home must therefore be seen as part of a larger project whereby the state used formal, public institutions to separate the needy and deviant from the rest of society. The influence of the Poor Law was important. These first institutions and those established later in the early decades of the twentieth century catered for a clientele that was equivalent to that of the workhouse and the workhouse infirmary.

Late nineteenth-century charitable homes for the aged have rightly been seen as a bridge between early poor law relief and the professionally administered, state-funded old age home of the twentieth century.[5] In contrast to regions of Canada and the United States with a longer history of non-aboriginal settlement and stable agrarian communities, however, there were few charitable old age homes in the western province before the 1940s. Nor did provincial municipalities follow the pattern that occurred elsewhere of building county workhouses where the indigent aged were sheltered along with unemployed, the sick, and the blind. The relatively sparse nature of urban settlement in B.C. hindered the development of local government services and middle-class philanthropic efforts.[6]

State old age homes did not continue their hold on public pride, no doubt another facet of the cultural heritage of the Poor Law. By the First World War institutions for the indigent elderly were regarded as distasteful necessities rather than fine civic virtues, not fitting easily alongside "worthwhile" state services like well-baby clinics and mothers' pensions. Nonetheless, the expansion of public facilities, which took place at both the provincial and municipal level, could not meet the increased demand for care, particularly for the infirm elderly. Two poor law institutional practices were in use in B.C. by the 1920s. Municipal administrators used private hospitals to "board out" elderly indigents in poor health. In Victoria and Vancouver, and in smaller towns across the province, public charges who were old and infirm were also kept in local hospitals. Meanwhile, government funding and a steady clientele of public patients encouraged expansion of private and charitable old age homes. As was the case elsewhere in Canada, Britain, and northern Europe, the state took a dynamic role in facilitating the expansion of residential accommodation for the aged.[7]

After the Second World War, the old age home was once again seen as a worthwhile social project. Moreover, a new appreciation for old age as a distinct phase in the life cycle fostered the development of architectural forms meant to meet the particular needs of older people. The elderly had metamorphosed into senior citizens who had fought a good war like the rest of the populace and now deserved compassionate care in their final years.

Thus, the old age home developed later in B.C. than elsewhere, with the provincial government taking a significant role in fostering institutional evolution. Successive political regimes established homes for the elderly, regulated private and philanthropic facilities, and prodded municipalities and charitable groups into providing residential accommodation for B.C.'s aged citizens.

This chapter charts institutional evolutions that reflect broader Canadian patterns and west coast peculiarities. Whenever possible, I try to provide descriptions of facilities and their surroundings: I want you to look around the building and then take a walk down the street. An aesthetic sensitivity to "setting" can help us understand the social and cultural "plot" contained in the narrative of the old age home. Our society's distaste for old age homes sometimes made this task difficult: the Vancouver Old People's Home existed for half a century, but was so poorly regarded that I could find no photographic image to use for descriptive purposes. There is just one photograph held in a public archive of the Victoria Old Men's Home and only a handful of images of private hospitals. In contrast, there are a number of good early images of the Provincial Home for Aged Men and a virtual cornucopia of press photographs of Victoria's beloved Home for Aged and Infirm Ladies (now Rose Manor).

The organization of this chapter is roughly chronological. I begin by outlining the early history of public institutions in B.C., then discuss the development of charitable and private accommodation for the aged in the first decades of the twentieth century. The third section examines state care in the 1940s and 1950s. I then look at private hospitals and charitable facilities in that same period.

EARLY PUBLIC INSTITUTIONAL PROVISION

The first period of institutional growth in B.C., which lasted from 1892 to the early 1920s, encompassed the establishment of two kinds of state residential care for elderly people. In the first instance, a small number of public facilities, primarily for able-bodied men, were set up. Overall, these new municipal and provincial institutions were seen as worthwhile civic enterprises. Often with farms or working gardens attached, and located outside the metropolis, they were designed as places of work rather than places of care, although their function changed as their inhabitants grew more infirm.

The second form of residential accommodation saw indigent old people, many of whom were in poor health, "hidden" in institutions that ostensibly cared for another clientele – the acutely ill, the disabled, or mothers and children. Before the 1940s, the presence of old people in such facilities was rarely commented upon. Institutional provision for this second group of old people was not imbued with the same sense of noble purpose that characterized civic old age homes of the time. Thus, these old people were "hidden" in both a physical and a cultural sense, shut out of public discourse and community perceptions of where and how the aged lived.

B.C's first two public old age homes were established for men, a reflection of the preponderance of single men among the aged poor of the province.[8] Both were civic facilities. In 1892 the City of Victoria opened an Old Men's Home in premises rented from the Royal Jubilee Hospital.[9] Two years later it moved to the Johnson House, a building owned by the city on the grounds of the Ross Bay Cemetery.[10] There were twenty-six inmates on New Year's Eve 1894.[11] For more than a decade the Old Men's Home and the cemetery jockeyed with each other for space until a new brick structure was constructed on an eleven and a half acre plot of land on the outskirts of the city.[12] Twenty-one inmates moved to the new premises in June of 1906, relieved to be off the grounds of the cemetery, at least temporarily.[13] By 1920 there were thirty-five residents in the Home.[14] That number rose to the maximum capacity of forty, and remained constant into the 1940s.

The new institution was situated on the edge of the city, reflecting the contemporary belief that homes for the aged should be established in a serene, pastoral setting.[15] A journalist of the period noted with approval the spacious grounds with fruit trees, flowers, and vegetable gardens. "The citizens visit the inmates," he continued, "bringing books and little comforts, and, above all, loving sympathy."[16] The journalist was careful to delineate between Victoria's new charitable venture and the poorhouse, but the earlier location on the grounds of the local cemetery must have underscored the low status of the inmates.

The Home was set back from Cadboro Bay Road, a main thoroughfare toward the outskirts of urban development. A new inmate of the 1930s, alighting from the streetcar that had carried him to his new

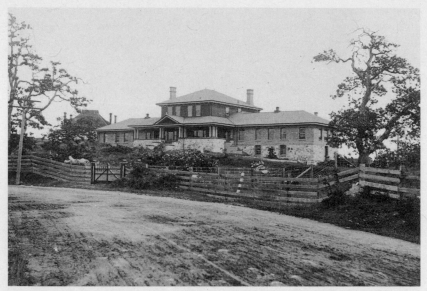

The Old Men's Home, Victoria, no date. Located on Cadboro Bay Road, outside the city limits but close to the Jubilee Hospital, the Home was built on a rocky outcrop of land in 1906 and remained in operation until it closed in 1962. The structure resembles a middle-class family home rather than an institution or grand civic enterprise. The house behind and to the left still stands, while the site of the Home is now occupied by Oak Bay Manor, a residential care facility for the elderly that opened in 1972 and was later renamed Oak Bay Lodge. (British Columbia Provincial Archives)

home, would have faced a substantial but unimposing brick building with a two-story central block flanked by two symmetrical wings. This kind of architecture, "derived" from the style of a family dwelling rather than "designed" as a grand public building, suggests a household rather than an institution.[17] Behind the Home lay a lower copse of garry oaks and broom and a rocky promontory with a wooden look-out giving views, on clear days, across the Straits of Juan de Fuca to Mount Baker. To the right was a block of arable land, which the city subdivided and sold off in 1951. The grounds were enclosed by a wooden fence.[18] This inmate would have slept in one of four large wards, with minimal privacy from other men provided by partitions that had been constructed in 1924.[19] If he became one of the institution's long-term inmates, surviving until 1951, he might have ended life in the new infirmary, added that year to accommodate the increasing numbers of infirm residents in the Home.[20]

The Provincial Home for Aged Men, built in 1894 in the interior town of Kamloops, had loftier institutional aspirations and a larger

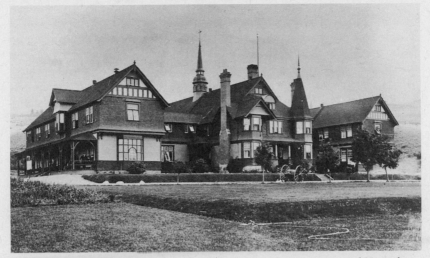

The Provincial Home for Aged Men, Kamloops, 1913. The 1894 Provincial Home for
Aged Men, which was in operation until 1975, was located close to the civic centre
of Kamloops. This photo shows the orginal central building, and two later flanking wings
in the Tudor Revival style. Note the cannon in front of the facility and the grand style
of the structure, an allusion to the social purpose of the province's haven for "pioneer
miners, trappers and lumbermen." Behind the dignified façade, however, conditions were
spartan, reinforcing the ethos of the poorhouse. (British Columbia Provincial Archives)

population. The purpose of the Home was "[t]o care for the old and
the infirm without suitable homes, particularly the pioneer miners,
trappers, lumbermen, and others who had opened up the new country
and were worn out in the struggle with nature ..."[21] Of the early public
homes for the aged in British Columbia, the Provincial Home was the
only one whose appearance presented a message of state charity as a
grand philanthropic enterprise. Only a few blocks from the business
centre of Kamloops, a broad, sweeping driveway brought the visitor
through well-kept grounds to the Home itself. Two newer wings in the
Tudor Revival style flanked the older central building. The Home was
kept in good condition, as was the Home Farm set to one side. Built
of the brick and frame construction common to public institutions of
the period, the Home was constructed for a clientele that was relatively
able-bodied.

The gracious public face of the building was not, however, duplicated inside. A spartan décor, the organization of space, and the institution's size – there were about 140 inmates by the 1930s – reflected
the lineage between the poorhouse and the public old age home.[22]
Administration and communal activities were conducted in the older

central unit, which was connected to two other buildings on each side
by a main hall or passageway. As was also the case at the Victoria Old
Men's Home, the superintendent's quarters were set above and apart
from the men's wards. An 1898 photograph shows a large cavernous
dining room with vaulted wooden ceilings and two long tables stretch-
ing the length of the room. There was another public room on the
second floor of the building, but it was used only for screening films
and was minimally furnished with just a few straight-backed chairs,
lacking even curtains or reading lamps. As architectural theorist
Thomas Markus notes, what is placed at the centre of a building is a
critical indication of its central purpose.[23] Institutional efficiency,
rather than comfort or sociability, was the organizing principle of the
Provincial Home's architecture and décor. No significant internal ren-
ovations were made until 1950, when the Home was "modernized"
by adding more lighting, plywood panelling, and white paint.[24]

Creature comforts were meagre and privacy limited. Residents appreciated the fact that they each had a small private room, described as a
"cubicle" in a 1941 report. In 1939 the curtains on these cubicles were
replaced with doors to give more privacy, and each man was assigned
a new bedside table, a freshly painted bed, and a chair.[25] One photograph from the Depression era shows a group of old men sitting on a
shaded back porch, likely the verandah built at the back of the hospital
ward in 1934 to give the inmates shelter from the hot summer sun.[26]

Over time, workhouse specifications were adapted to suit a more
frail clientele. There had always been a space for ill inmates, but a
report from the 1940s details a new sick bay that had been set up in
a former auditorium on the north side of the building. The Poor Law
ethos continued to prevail, despite the institutional acknowledgment
that this space was for patients, not inmates. The two sick bays served
twenty-six patients, but had only three toilets and one open bath.
There were no call bells, draw curtains, or bed lights.[27]

We know less about the physicality of the Old People's Home in
Vancouver, although the history of its establishment is in itself an
illustration of how the impoverished elderly were housed wherever
space could be found. The municipal Home was built in 1915 to
accommodate a group of aged paupers, all men, who had been living
since 1900 in the old buildings of the General Hospital at the intersection of Pender and Cambie streets. The hospital moved to new
premises at Fairview Heights in 1905, leaving approximately seventeen
"poor old people" behind. These men were in varying stages of health.
Some, though not acutely ill, had been institutionalized for more than
five years. The more able-bodied assisted with chores around the hospital, sawing firewood, sorting laundry, and delivering messages. Aged

indigents were also housed in the old civic jail and at the crematory caretaker's house.[28]

Pressure grew to provide a home for the city's aged indigents, and in 1915 forty-five men and women moved into a new two-story brick structure two blocks south of Hastings Street at Cassiar Street and Boundary Road. The entire site was forty acres in total and had been logged only ten years previously.[29] This location was a good walk from the eastern terminus of the No. 20 streetcar, which ran through the Vancouver waterfront and into the nexus of the city's male working-class life.[30] Prospective residents from the old hospital, who, it was charged, wandered the streets of Vancouver drunk, were thus removed from the busy commercial and respectable residential areas.[31]

Newspaper accounts lauded the "sunny surroundings" and "up-to-date" kitchen arrangements of the new facility that replaced the unsuitably "dingy quarters" of the hospital.[32] Its accommodation for couples was rare in public facilities,[33] and it was the first state institution in the young province to provide accommodation for elderly women. Yet the use of patient labour in an institution that was apparently run as a farm in its early years, the means-tested entrance qualifications, and the dominance of male inmates meant that this new facility in fact had much in common with its institutional peers in Kamloops and Victoria. The Home was administered by the City Health Department until 1936, when it was placed under the direction of the City Relief Department.

The Old People's Home was bigger than Victoria's civic Home, with a population of approximately sixty inmates throughout the 1930s. The main floor of the building had a kitchen, dining room, two public rooms, and eight sleeping rooms, one of which contained eight beds and the others either two beds or one. The largest ward, with space for sixteen inmates, was on the second floor, alongside five smaller rooms. Elderly women, always fewer in number than men, occupied the north wing of the ground floor. In 1914 thirty-two men and two women were resident at the Home. In 1930 there were fifty men and twelve women. Prospective residents, driven to enter the Home because they had no other means of subsistence, would have had their misfortune and vulnerability underscored by the cheerless conditions of bare wooden floors, dark woodwork, and buff-coloured walls. Before a 1945 redecorating effort, the Home had dormitories where "a single bare light bulb glared from the centre of the ceiling and white beds with white coverlets stood mutely side by side." The few single rooms at the Vancouver facility were awarded on the basis of seniority, which meant that one would await the death of a fellow resident with mixed feelings.[34]

Institutions like Kamloops' Provincial Home and civic facilities in Vancouver and Victoria were founded specifically as homes for the aged and based on the Poor Law idea that inmates would be able-bodied and capable of working for their keep. The infirm and chronically ill were "hidden" elsewhere. The Provincial Home for Incurables, which later became the Marpole branch of the Provincial Infirmary system, was located in the Marpole district of Vancouver and acquired by the province from the Vancouver General Hospital in 1923, and it functioned as a workhouse infirmary rather than a workhouse itself.[35] As the sorry name of the institution makes clear, the Home was to serve no grand social purpose, but was regarded as a dumping ground for the most hopeless poor of the province. Most of its residents were elderly indigents with chronic health problems. There was no expectation that these people would work for their keep.

An institution that could make no claim to social improvement did not deserve a purpose-built structure or a countrified location. The Marpole facility had begun life as the Grand Hotel, built in 1913 at the corner of busy South West Marine Drive and Hudson Street, on the border between areas of residential dwellings and light industry. The brick façade rose four stories: bed patients were housed on the first two floors, ambulatory patients on the third floor, and staff on the fourth. There was an interior garden with wheelchair access, but most patients preferred to spend time outside the front of the institution, chatting with passersby and observing the activities of the area. A close look at the photo of the Home shows several wheelchairs on the sidewalk in front.

Plagued by persistent rumours of closure, building maintenance at the Home for Incurables was neglected and the institution's interior was drab and dark. Space was extremely limited: the cafeteria was actually underneath the sidewalk outside the building. Even the morgue doubled as a room for sorting laundry for a time. The rooms here were larger than at any other public institution in the province, with the biggest containing thirty-three beds for men. On the women's wards, a hint of colour was provided by a rose-coloured blanket folded at the foot of each bed, a gift of the Women's Auxiliary at the institution.[36]

Inmates at the Home were part of a large and complex institutional community. Twenty-three women and ninety-nine men were admitted during the first year the facility was operated by the provincial government. By 1930 the patient population had increased to 180, and the seven staff included a superintendent who was a medical doctor, a matron who was a registered nurse, a bursar or clerk, and four nurses. In this early period care was purely custodial, with a range of patients from ambulatory to bedridden. A decade later there were sixty

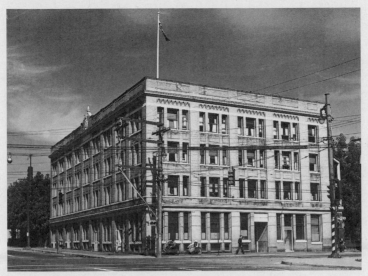

The Provincial Home for Incurables (Marpole Infirmary), Vancouver, ca 1950.
A later photo of the Vancouver branch of the Provincial Infirmary. Built in 1913
as a hotel and taken over by the province a decade later, the facility is an
example of a "borrowed" building that was ill-suited for the infirm aged.
Many residents, however, appreciated the urban milieu of the facility, preferring
to spend time out on the busy street corner rather than in the internal
garden. This facility closed in 1965. (British Columbia Provincial Archives)

staff and an energetic Women's Auxiliary to take care of the needs of
a smaller patient population of 159. This shift in staff-patient ratios
reflects a new interest in chronic illness and rehabilitative medicine.[37]

The case of the Sannich Health Centre, constructed in 1920 in the
agricultural municipality bordering on Victoria, is another illustration
of how old people found accommodation in a range of institutions.
The centre was built as a tribute to the men and women who were
involved in the war effort, and as a gesture of hope that a better society
would emerge from the conflict. In its first decade it served as the nexus
for an ambitious public health program that included health inspections of school children, maternity work, infant welfare, and tonsil and
tuberculosis clinics. Although elderly people are not mentioned in a
1925 pamphlet promoting the centre, from the early years they were
accommodated on the top floor of the building.[38]

By 1932 the Corporation of Saanich had rented the centre out to
Ruth C. Thomson as a private hospital caring primarily for elderly
public patients. In 1940 Miss Jane Nixon became the manager of
the centre, by then renamed the Royal Oak Private Hospital, paying

forty dollars per month for the use of the premises. Nixon, in turn, charged the municipality forty dollars per month for each ambulatory case and forty-five to fifty dollars per month for each bed case, depending upon the amount of care required. Twenty elderly men slept on the ground floor and ten women made use of the second floor. Nixon continued to run the facility until 1952, when she turned her license over to Mr and Mrs Emery.[39]

Instead of creating public old age homes for the infirm elderly, municipal governments in Vancouver and Victoria made formal agreements with local hospitals to care for these people. The Vancouver General Hospital housed the chronically ill in several locations, including the future Home for Incurables and two wooden frame annexes that had been originally constructed for wounded veterans and Spanish influenza patients. By 1928 there were 250 chronic patients at the 12th Avenue Annex. The Annex was moved to 13th Avenue and Willow Street and licensed as a private hospital in 1948. This institution cared for elderly chronically ill male patients.[40] The City of Victoria made formal arrangements with the Jubilee Hospital and St Joseph's Hospital in 1925 to care for indigent patients at a set monthly rate. The agreement with the Jubilee Hospital continued until 1938, by which time the City of Victoria was paying $700 per month for this service.[41]

These arrangements were scarcely revolutionary, for B.C.'s hospitals had been used for the infirm and indigent elderly since they were first established. The original residents of Vancouver's Old People's Home were displaced hospital patients. St Joseph's Hospital, established in Victoria in 1876 by the Sisters of Saint Ann, had an old men's ward.[42] Inmates at Victoria's Old Men's Home were routinely moved to the nearby Jubilee Hospital when they became seriously ill.[43] These practices were linked in the public mind to an older idea of charitable hospitals for the poor.[44] Perhaps, as a provincial bureaucrat later suggested, this process enabled the aged infirm and their families to avoid the stigma attached to public welfare institutions such as the Provincial Home for Aged Men.[45] This option was attractive to municipalities as well, for provincial hospital grants were paid on the basis of occupied beds.

But the use of local hospital beds to accommodate elderly indigents generated tension for a number of reasons. Hospital administrators were uneasy about caring for this group of patients. In 1924 George McGregor, the president of Victoria's Jubilee Hospital, stated that he did not want the Jubilee "used as an old men's or old women's home." The agreement reached the following year with the City of Victoria allayed fears about the local hospital becoming a dumping ground for aged indigents, but Jubilee Hospital administrators were never particularly happy with the arrangement. Nor was the provincial government content to continue funding municipal hospital patients. As early as 1930 the provincial government was formulating plans to force municipalities to take more responsibility for indigent patients in local hospitals.[46]

As the case of Miss Jane Nixon and the Saanich Health Centre shows, another way that municipalities dealt with the problem of infirm indigents was to pay for their keep in private hospitals. From 1922 welfare administrators in Victoria placed patients from the Jubilee Hospital and the Old Men's Home who were sick but did not require acute hospital care in the Maple Rest Nursing Home and another private facility on Blanchard Street.[47] Before it began leasing out its former health centre for use as a private hospital, Saanich municipality also sent bed patients to the Maple Rest Nursing Home and to at least one other institution, the Dalkeith Nursing Home.[48] During the same period City of Vancouver welfare administrators also began placing elderly public charges in private hospitals, such as the Glen, Grandview, and Bayview hospitals.[49] Officials found that this practice reduced hospital overcrowding and saved public funds. City administrators in Victoria, for example, paid the Jubilee Hospital $2.50 per diem for indigent patients in 1920. Four years later the health officer noted that the Maple Rest and Blanchard Street homes were charging the city only $1.33 per patient per day.[50]

The limited development of public old age homes in B.C. in its first decades of sustained non-aboriginal settlement was mostly the result of settlement patterns and the provincial economy: by the First World War, B.C. did not have the municipal resources and community structures to create a system of local workhouses as could be found in Ontario and the Maritimes. Instead, two patterns emerged. First, the provincial state took on a strong role as an innovator and a provider of residential care for both the able-bodied and the infirm indigent elderly of the province. The model for the two provincial institutions and the two municipal old age homes established during this early period was clearly the poorhouse or the workhouse infirmary. Second, local hospitals and private establishments took a formal role in the care of old people who were sick and unable to pay for their keep. Not publicly identified as homes for the aged, these should be regarded as "hidden" old age homes.

EARLY PHILANTHROPIC
AND PRIVATE OLD AGE HOMES

The early history of charitable old age homes and private hospital accommodation for the elderly in the western province reflected the peculiarities of B.C.'s social and political structures. Only three philanthropic facilities existed before 1940, an indication of the limited nature of charitable organization in the province. These institutions, two of which were for Chinese men and one for "respectable" European women, developed in response to specific gaps in state care rather than as independent charitable efforts to care for the aged. As I have noted, private care for old people also evolved in response to the needs of the state: the use of small independent hospitals for public municipal patients became common in Vancouver and Victoria in the inter-war years. Operators of these facilities, responding to a changing market of care provision, shifted their focus from maternity and surgical care to the provision of medical and convalescent nursing – a patient category that appears to have included a large number of elderly people.

Although the City of Victoria had established its Old Men's Home in the late nineteenth century, the municipal council refused to build a similar facility for old women. Like other middle-class women who created homes for the elderly across North America during the same period, the women who founded the Home for Aged and Infirm Ladies were motivated by a sense of religious duty and a belief that the respectable impoverished gentlewomen of the city were a deserving clientele.[51] In 1897 they rented the hospital premises that had been used five years previously by the Old Men's Home. In 1908 a new building with thirty-five bedrooms, a large dining room, a concert hall, and a sunroom was constructed with financial assistance from the City of Victoria and the Province of British Columbia. The gracious front façade of the building, with curved arches and a rooftop cupola, speaks to the institution's genteel public image.[52]

Three years after the new building was completed, a wing was added using funds donated by the provincial and municipal governments and friends of the Home. By 1912 the Home was large enough to house between seventy and eighty women, more than twice the population at the new civic facility for men.[53] In 1947 there were 113 female residents and a staff of thirty. A 1948 newspaper editorial described the institution as a "fine block of brick and stone buildings fronting on McClure and Rupert Streets. To the passerby it looks like a well-appointed hotel, but to the inmates it really is a home, with all that name implies."[54]

The physical organization of space and community at the Home for Aged and Infirm Ladies echoed this theme of the old age home as hotel, demonstrating a much greater regard for comfort and aesthetic niceties than was evident across town at the Old Men's Home. Although the women living in the Home did help out with kitchen chores, the building and grounds were not laid out with that purpose in mind. Let us

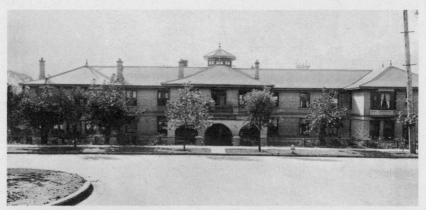

The Home for Aged and Infirm Ladies (Rose Manor), Victoria, 1920s. This venerable Victoria institution still operates as a home for the elderly. The well-kept gardens, roof-top cupola, and gracious façade of the building hint at the respectable position that the 1908 facility occupied in civic charitable circles. Private patients occupied the front rooms, with views out to the treed residential street, while public patients were housed in rooms overlooking St Joseph's Catholic Hospital. (British Columbia Provincial Archives)

accompany an incoming resident of 1940 into her new home. We walk from Rupert Street up to the main door through a medley of one hundred rose bushes, donated by the municipal park superintendent the previous year and the future inspiration for the name "Rose Manor," adopted in 1950. We are greeted by Miss Alice Robb, the valued matron with a soft Scottish accent. Passing through the dining room where framed portraits of the Home's founders are hung, the new resident is shown the chapel, the sunrooms, and the sitting rooms. A private rather than a public patient, our friend will find her room, overlooking the front gardens and the street, furnished with her own bed, chest of drawers, and armchair. Returning to the dining room for lunch, she will sit at an intimate table with five other women, a contrast to the long crowded benches used by men at the Provincial Home. She could as easily have checked into a hotel of quality as entered an old age home.[55]

The divide between public and private patients at the Victoria institution seems to have stopped at the doors to their personal rooms. All residents benefited from the pains taken by the Home Management Committee over the exterior and interior décor of the building. In 1936, for example, the committee personally selected flowers for Christmas to decorate the Home. The committee was always involved in selecting linens, draperies, and floor coverings for the Home: at the February meeting in 1937, for instance, samples of bath towels and face clothes were considered and a special meeting called a few days later to look at linoleum patterns. In 1949 Miss Boulton, the matron, brought samples of china to show the committee, and a rose pattern was selected.[56] This emphasis on gentility reflected institutional pride, the presence of paying guests within the Home, the class background of the institution's administrators, and gendered assumptions about the sensibilities of elderly women.

As the history of the Home's expansion makes evident, the financial base of the facility was a combination of money from private and municipal patients and investment income in legacies from appreciative residents and members of the local elite. In 1937, for instance, a generous legacy of $2,000, from Mrs L.M. Dunsmuir, a member of the one of the province's early entrepreneurial and political families, covered some of the construction costs of a new wing.[57] The institution took in both private and public cases, and charged rates based on the level of care required and the standard of accommodation provided. State support was critical, both in the provision of money for new building projects and in ensuring a guaranteed income from public patients. Funds from the City of Victoria and Saanich municipality brought a steady revenue into the institutional coffers. The seventeen public patients in 1923 cost the City of Victoria $4,912.50. By 1928 the number of public patients had risen to thirty and the amount charged for their care to $6,714.05.[58] Occasionally, other municipalities – Vancouver, New Westminster, or Kamloops, for example – also sent public patients to the facility.[59]

In contrast to the assured income that public patients brought, collecting money from private patients was sometimes more difficult. Long periods of institutional care depleted the savings of many women who entered the Home as paying residents. In 1926, for example, Amelia Whittier, secretary-treasurer for the Home Committee, petitioned the City of Victoria to pay for the keep of two spinster sisters, Elsbeth and Amelia Travis. The Travis sisters, aged seventy-five and sixty-five, had entered the Home four years previously as private patients. By 1926, however, the legacy left to them by a deceased judge had been exhausted and they were forced to turn to public funds.[60]

Monthly meetings of the Home Management Committee always began with silent prayer and moved on to careful discussions of institutional finance and management. Men were entirely absent from the operation of the home. Representing a cross-section of religious organizations in the city, the women of the board were astute administrators and able politicians, using their links to local elites to solicit funds and support for the Home.[61] For example, a 1901 interview with Mayor Hayward, whose wife was a past president of the committee, secured a commitment that the city solicitor would undertake any business required by the Home and that the chief of the police would assist with a difficult inmate.[62]

A remarkable administrative continuity within the Home ensured institutional stability. Daughters and other female relations took over the committee work done by the previous generation. Amelia Whittier, daughter of Harriet Carne, a founding committee member, joined the Home Committee in 1917 and served as secretary-treasurer from 1920 to 1943. She was elected president from 1946 to 1948.[63] When Mrs McTavish, an early committee member, resigned in 1921, Mrs Clay, the president of the committee, noted that she was glad that McTavish had been replaced by Mrs Heddle, a connection of the McTavish family.[64] Elite networks, a strong sense of religious duty, and careful administration characterized the work of these women.

Victoria's Chinese Consolidated Benevolent Association also became involved in providing residential accommodation for the aged during the late nineteenth century, responding to the terrible circumstances of the indigent elderly men in their community. As was the case with the Home for Aged and Infirm Ladies, the institution was created for a specific community of elderly people. The predominance of single men among Victoria's Chinese community during this period is striking, but Chinese men were not permitted to enter the Old Men's Home or the Provincial Home in Kamloops.[65] In 1884 the association rented a small wooden hut and established a *Tiapinfang* (small hospital) for ailing indigent men. Five years later the association was able to purchase a lot on Herald Street and build the Zhonghua Yiyuan (Chinese Hospital), a two-story brick edifice.[66]

Here again, there is a pattern of unwillingness on the part of the state to provide care balanced by a tacit acknowledgment of the necessity of government support for the ongoing existence of charitable enterprise. In the 1920s the hospital, facing serious financial problems, underwent an evolution from independent charity to state-subsidized and -supported facility. Institutional revenues dropped as it became more difficult to collect compulsory donations from Chinese men returning to their homeland. Costs rose when the City of Victoria decided to collect taxes on the hospital property. A shrinking Chinese population, coupled with a growing acceptance of Western medicine, meant that the Chinese Consolidated Benevolent Association no longer saw the operation of the hospital as crucial within the Chinese community. In 1929 the City took possession of the hospital property because of unpaid taxes and leased it back to the association for a monthly rent of thirty dollars. From this point onward the City of Victoria played an active role in ensuring the continued existence of the Chinese Hospital. Civic welfare administrators apparently thought it was cheaper to maintain an existing facility than find a new place to house the hospital residents.[67]

With financial and administrative support from the City of Victoria and an ongoing clientele of elderly male Chinese-Canadian public patients, the Chinese Hospital was able to consolidate its position during the 1930s. In 1938, the city granted the hospital a monthly sum of fifty dollars and an additional ten dollars per month for each patient. Two years later Dr Richard Felton, the city medical officer, took on the additional role of superintendent at the institution.[68] The Chinese Consolidated Benevolent Association opened a new twenty-bed hospital in the heart of Chinatown in 1942.[69] Patient statistics from the 1950s and early 1960s indicate that the hospital was providing both convalescent and long-term care. In February 1963 approval was granted for a concrete extension with thirteen new beds, a nurse's station, a patient's lounge, and a new main entrance.[70]

A society called the "Chinese Old Man's Home of New Westminster, B.C." also existed during the early twentieth century, although it is not clear how long it was in operation or if a residential facility was actually established. The society was first incorporated in 1913 and was still active in 1926. Among the eight directors listed in the society's 1926 bylaws, six were merchants, one was a labourer, and the other a cook. Funding for the Home was based on a yearly subscription fee of one dollar.[71] In Vancouver during the 1940s, St Joseph's Oriental Hospital cared for thirty-five chronically ill Chinese men on its top floor, most of whom were elderly.[72]

While there were a few charitable homes for the aged, private hospitals took an increasing number of elderly patients, both private and public, during the inter-war years. With maternity and surgical cases now being cared for in the expanding general hospital, private hospitals evolved toward the care of the chronically ill, the convalescent, and the aged. By the 1930s the business of providing medical and convalescent care was becoming more economically feasible than nursing expectant mothers and young babies.[73] Most private hospitals were small, somewhat marginal institutions run independently by women. In 1934, for example, five of the seven private hospitals in Victoria had fewer than ten patient beds. Ownership and location of these institutions was often fluid.[74]

The use of private hospitals by municipal welfare administrators created new business opportunities for the proprietors of B.C.'s private hospitals. Larger private hospitals were invariably those that took public patients. In 1934, Victoria's Maple Rest Nursing Home, the largest private hospital in the city, had twenty-four beds, which were mostly occupied by city patients too frail to enter the Old Men's Home or the Home for Aged and Infirm Ladies.[75] In Vancouver, public patients went to the Grandview, Glen, Bayview, Royal Derby, and Florence Nightingale hospitals, providing a steady source of revenue for their proprietors. Miss Kate Smith, a graduate nurse, opened the Glen Hospital with her sister Mrs Mary Westwood in 1920 with only four beds. By 1937, however, with the assurance of a steady income from public patients, the family institution had expanded to eighty-six beds.[76]

These early private hospitals, located in older residential dwellings that were marginally remodelled for their new purpose, bore little resemblance to the modern general hospital that was then emerging. Glen Hospital, at the corner of Salisbury and Napier streets, was located in the former home of an Australian millionaire, although a modern concrete annex was added in 1937.[77] Vancouver's Grandview Hospital was described in the 1950s as "a very large old house," in "run down condition."[78] Descriptions of the interiors of these places are rare, but the 1933 investigation into the Maple Rest Nursing Home in Victoria found that some of the sixteen patients were housed in the basement of the facility with, as two indignant aldermen claimed, "insufficient light and ventilation to meet the requirements of the by-law governing the stabling of a cow." There was apparently only one bathroom for the use of the entire patient population, and it was located on the second floor.[79]

Private hospitals and charitable old age homes filled an important niche in the care of B.C.'s elderly in the early twentieth century. Of these two kinds of institutions, it is evident that the most dynamic growth ocurred among the small-scale capitalist endeavours of nursing homes like the Maple Rest in Victoria or the Grandview in Vancouver. The first philanthropic homes for the elderly in the province were created in response to specific gaps in state provision, not as part of a larger trend toward charitable residential care for deserving citizens. Both kinds of institutions relied on money from the state.

STATE FACILITIES IN THE 1940S AND 1950S

In British Columbia, the 1940s and 1950s were decades of shifting state engagement with institutional provision for the aged. Expansion of provincial facilities was piecemeal, motivated by a relentless demand for accommodation, but municipalities began to take a more innovative and dynamic role, renovating existing buildings and constructing

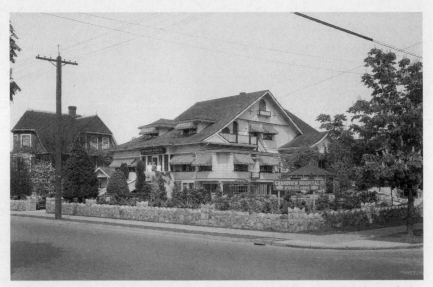

Grandview Hospital and Nursing Home, Vancouver, 1940s. A rare image of one of Vancouver's largest private hospitals during the 1940s. Grandview, with sixty beds at the time this picture was taken, was larger than most private hospitals in the city. Grandview was nonetheless typical of many private hospitals of this period with its location in a recycled family dwelling and in its increasing reliance on public patients and the elderly. (Stuart Thomson photo, City of Vancouver Archives CVA 99-4891)

new facilities with an elderly clientele in mind. Although hampered by the dearth of construction materials following the Second World War, a new architectural model for the old age home was emerging. The province, in contrast, attempted to limit its role as a provider of institutional facilities for the aged,[80] using new funding programs to encourage both municipal and voluntary schemes.

The establishment of Mount Saint Mary's Hospital in Victoria in the early 1940s, a branch of the Provincial Infirmary system, demonstrates the new arms-length relationship that the provincial government favoured in regard to institutions for the aged. In 1941 the Liberal government formed a partnership with the Sisters of Saint Ann, granting the order $50,000 to help cover construction costs of the new facility. In return, the Sisters agreed to provide care for 100 public bed cases.[81] In this fashion, the province channelled public patients into an institution that was run by a reputable charitable group rather than by the state.

This was the first B.C. institution designed and built for a specific clientele of infirm elderly. It was also the first old age home to be constructed in the province since the Vancouver Old People's Home

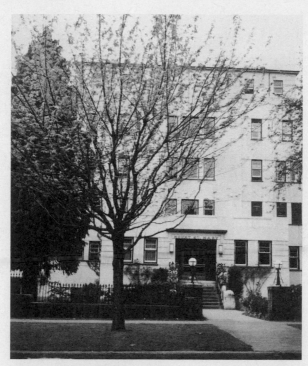

Mount Saint Mary's Hospital, Victoria, 1943. Constructed in
1941 with joint funding from the Sisters of Saint Ann and the
provincial government, Mount Saint Mary's was the first old
age home in B.C. designed and built specifically for a clientele
of infirm elderly. Three stories high and constructed of light
stone, the style of the building resembles a modern hospital,
reflecting a desire to link the old age home to the hospital
ethos of efficiency, sanitation, and bureaucatic functionalism.
(British Columbia Provincial Archives)

was completed in 1916, and the functional evolution of residential
accommodation for the aged from poor law institution to health care
facility was clearly evident. Located in a quiet semi-residential street
across from the Anglican cathedral, the Catholic institution resembled
a modern hospital, office block, or apartment building. The building's
style, coupled with its location away from Victoria's commercial and
social clusters, discouraged interaction between elderly patients and
the larger community. Residents of the new building were meant to be
ill, not integrated members of the local neighbourhood.

Architecturally, Mount Saint Mary's was a clear departure from the
familial style of the municipal Old Men's Home and the esteemed
social purpose of the Home for Aged and Infirm Ladies or the Provincial

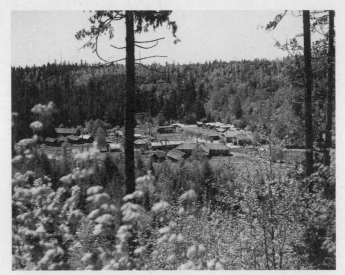

Allco Provincial Infirmary, Fraser Valley, 1920s. This picture of Allco
Provincial Infirmary, a former logging camp and relief camp hospital,
is another illustration of how recycled institutions were used for the
aged. The camp, located five miles east of Haney in B.C.'s Fraser
Valley and made up a collection of small wooden cabins, was totally
unsuited for elderly men in uncertain health, yet it operated as such
from 1943 to 1964. (British Columbia Provincial Archives)

Home. Three stories high and built of light stone, its striking resemblance to the 1935 tuberculosis wing of the Vancouver General Hospital reflected a new desire to link institutional geriatic care to the
twentieth-century hospital and its ambience of efficiency, sanitation,
and bureaucratic functionalism. Experts in hospital administration
praised its clean, modern appearance and noted with appreciation the
smaller wards, which came closer to meeting the ideal of patient privacy. The construction of private rooms for paying patients, in addition
to shared public facilities, was another nod to the modern hospital.[82]
    But the opening of Mount Saint Mary's did not herald a complete
shift from workhouse accommodation to hospital care for B.C.'s infirm
aged. Nor did the new facility alleviate the demand for space within
the Provincial Infirmary system. Two years later another branch of the
system, described as "one of Canada's strangest and most primitive
hospitals," was established in a remote forested area five miles east of
Haney on the Allouette River.[83] This institution certainly failed to
conform to any current thought concerning appropriate accommodation for the aged. Administrators rationalized the use of Allco, a

former logging camp and relief hospital, by maintaining that it was appropriate for men who had spent their lives in the bush. In fact, the institution was totally unsuitable for elderly people in uncertain health. Allco was another "hidden" institution, a place where old men considered too rough to be housed in an urban milieu would be set apart from society.[84] Its use demonstrates the durability of poor law attitudes toward the impoverished aged and the very low status of single old men on the margins of B.C. society.

Travelling to the camp through the surrounding forest, an inmate of the 1940s might well have believed that he was decades younger and taking up a new work assignment at some isolated logging outfit. Photographic images of the period show a cluster of small wooden cabins, about twenty-five in total, in the midst of scrub bush and conifers. The eighty male inmates at Allco slept with two or three other men in the original loggers' shacks. Accommodation in these small huts was certainly rough: heated by cheap wood stoves, only half of the cabins had indoor plumbing. The other facilities were each housed in separate buildings, including washrooms, a dining room, a sitting room, a kitchen, and the doctor's office and dispensary. Wet and cold weather was particularly hazardous as the old men struggled to reach the toilet or dining room.[85]

Municipal developments were more enterprising during this period. In 1943, Victoria's Post-War Rehabilitation Committee recommended that a 200-bed old age home be established when the war ended, and also considered financing construction of cottage homes for the elderly. But work began on the facility even before the close of the war, pushed ahead by a 1944 Victoria Council of Social Agencies study that found that sixty-six elderly patients in St Joseph's and the Royal Jubilee hospitals could be discharged to a nursing home if such a facility were opened. City administrators first attempted to interest the neighbouring municipalities of Esquimalt, Oak Bay, and Saanich in a joint venture, but in the end established the Victoria Nursing Home by themselves.[86]

The Victoria Nursing Home, run by a society of the same name, opened in 1945 with twenty-one beds.[87] Its first institutional home was the imposing, ivy-covered former residence of Emily Dunsmuir, the fifth daughter of coal magnate Robert Dunsmuir. Disused military facilities, no longer required once the war years had passed, were also converted into residential accommodation for the elderly.[88] In the Fraser Valley, Chilliwack's former military hospital became Valley Haven in 1948, home for sixteen men and twenty-two women. Here, some privacy was provided for the elderly women residents by curtains that divided their bedrooms. Male residents were "proud possessors of small individual rooms."[89] A similar scheme to convert the Tillicum

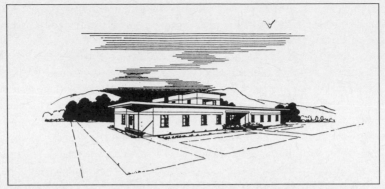

David Lloyd-Jones Home, Kelowna, 1949. This post-Second World War
municipal old age home, built in the largest town in the Okanagan region,
represents the new ideas behind residential accommodation for seniors that
dominated by the 1950s. Presenting features reminiscent of both hospital and
"home," such facilities attempted to convey a dualistic image of competent
scientific professionalism and home-like family care. The low-rise design was
characteristic of public and private institutions contructed for elderly people
in the 1950s and 1960s. (*Kelowna Courier*, 21 July 1949)

Army Camp was considered by the municipality of Saanich, but
rejected as being too costly.[90]

A small number of municipalities, like Saanich, held fast to the argument that they were not responsible for providing residential accommodation for their senior citizens.[91] Yet overall, the 1940s and 1950s
saw dynamic growth in municipal old age homes in B.C. Civic administrators placed these facilities high on their list of post-war reconstruc-
tion projects: Nelson, Prince Rupert, New Westminster, Langley, Surrey,
Courtney, and Kelowna all established some form of residential accommodation for elderly men and women in their communities, likely using
building grants from the provincial government.

By the late 1940s, purpose-built municipal homes for aged British
Columbians had begun to open. Pioneer Home was established in
Prince Rupert in 1946. Five years later Kelowna's new David Lloyd-
Jones Home opened with space for twenty-eight elderly city residents.
In 1954 the Dunsmuir residence was demolished to make way for a
modern, purpose-built structure and the Victoria Nursing Home was
renamed the Gorge Road Hospital. The cost of the nursing home was
paid for in part by a grant from the provincial government.[92]

Architecturally, these new facilities mixed features of both hospital
and "home," attempting to convey a dualistic image of competent,

scientific professionalism and home-like, family care. New, purpose-built old age homes, like the David Lloyd-Jones Home, were built with nursing stations and other medical facilities. The design of these homes, with rooms facing toward an inner courtyard, emphasized the fact that the old age home was regarded as separate from the larger community.

Newly built old age homes had communal sitting rooms and a larger number of bathrooms, both of which were undoubtedly appreciated by their residents. However, shared rather than single rooms continued to be customary at both old and new facilities. As one welfare worker wrote in 1950, it was hard to gauge the effect of the loss of privacy and independence. However, the importance of personal space in the old age home could be judged by "the evident satisfaction of the old lady in a room of her own who points with pride to the small personal possessions which so frequently 'clutter up' her small domain."[93]

The province's attempts to recycle Allco, an older facility, and to contract out care to the respectable Sisters of Saint Ann, while having historical precedents – the Provincial Home for Incurables had started life as the Grand Hotel and local and private hospitals had long been used for public patients – illustrate the government's desire to limit its involvement in the provision of residential accommodation for elderly people, and demonstrate the low status of the aged on the provincial policy agenda.

In general, by the post-war period, municipalities proved willing to take on the role of creating institutions for the elderly, albeit with assistance from provincial coffers. The renovation of older buildings in the 1940s and the construction of new municipal old age homes in the 1950s were very much features of the post-war municipal social agenda in British Columbia. Two models of design emerged in public old age homes of the period – the old age home as hospital and the old age home as a middle-class family dwelling. The case of Allco, however, shows how poor law models persisted even in a time of change. But regardless of whether the ideas were new or old, the architecture and location of public institutions closed off the old age home from the local community.

PHILANTHROPIC AND PRIVATE OLD AGE HOMES AND THE WELFARE STATE

Private and charitable old age homes in B.C. grew substantially in size and in number during the 1940s and 1950s. From 1947 provincial government grants were available to assist charitable agencies wishing to build residential accommodation for the elderly, and ethnic and religious groups responded with enthusiasm. In general, however, these groups created institutions for ambulatory patients rather than the more costly facilities required for bed patients. As was the case with public institutions, old age homes were established both in older buildings adapted for the elderly and in purpose-built structures. The prospect of a steady stream of public patients provided another financial boost to charitable old age homes, private hospitals, and boarding homes. Particularly in the years following the Second World War, the extreme shortage of private hospital beds meant that such establishments were able to charge high rates and expand their operations substantially.[94]

Even before provincial funding made such enterprises more economically feasible, philanthropic organizations in B.C. were becoming interested in the old age home. The post-war housing shortage meant that older frame and stone family homes were converted for use by the aged. With little ground floor accommodation, these residences were ill-suited to the elderly infirm, although they usually had attractive and sizeable grounds. A wealthy Vancouver widow, for example, bought and renovated a "rambling" Georgia Street mansion that had belonged to the B.C. sugar magnate B.T. Rogers. Twenty-five old men were resident there in 1946.[95]

Religious groups moved into the institutional care of the elderly during the 1940s. By 1944 a number of ecumenical organizations were reporting to the provincial Welfare Institutions Board, the government agency responsible for residential accommodation for the ambulatory aged. In Vancouver, St Jude's Home for the Aged had twenty-two beds while St Vincent's Home and Shelter had space for fifty-six people. Some old people also resided at the Convent of the Good Shepherd. In Victoria, an order of Anglican Sisters called the Society for the Love of Jesus opened Saint Mary's Priory with seventy-four beds in 1943. In 1951 the Salvation Army opened Sunset Lodge, which housed thirty-two "guests" in its first year. In addition, two other religious institutions were listed as boarding homes in the provincial capital: Saint Mary's Home, with eleven beds, and the Rainbow Christian Fellowship, with space for eight people.[96]

Victoria's Caroline Macklem Home, established by the Anglican Church, was one charitable old age home established in a "borrowed" family dwelling. Part of a larger ecumenical effort for Victoria's seniors, the Home's founding was made possible by a large financial bequest and the 1950 donation of Shulhuum, a substantial Victorian Tudor Revival building in the affluent Rockland area of the city.[97] The Home was for women only and preference was given to Anglican applicants. The religious base of the facility was underscored through daily prayer in institution's chapel. By 1953 there were twenty-four residents. It must have been unsettling to live in a place so replete with icons testifying to the grandeur of its former owners. Early records note the grand piano, luxurious rugs, and beautiful tapestries and drapes left by the owner, while lamenting the lack of ground floor rooms and a sick bay for ailing residents.[98] As Peter Townsend noted in his seminal study of old age homes in England and Wales, the "ornamental excesses" of such wealthy homes might well have been disconcerting, even frightening, for the new residents.[99]

Nelson's Mount St Francis, opened by the Sisters of Saint Ann in the same year as the Caroline Macklem Home, followed a different pattern of development. The establishment of the new Kootenay facility demonstrates the high cost of providing facilities and caring for bed patients and indicates a shift toward purpose-built old age homes in B.C. An initial scheme to use the original ranch house on the McKim estate was eventually replaced by a plan to construct a costly new fireproof building with space for seventy-five aged men and women. A staff of five sisters and twenty-seven paid employees ran the new facility and cared for the residents, most of whom were non-ambulatory. Funds for the new institution came from the federal and provincial governments, the Sisters, the public, and the Consolidated Mining and Smelting Company, who were induced to provide for the "poor exhausted, broken bodies of our pioneers in the late evening of their colourful lives."[100] The high level of state funding meant that the Sisters were obliged to meet numerous government criteria for building codes and patient selection, but they were eager to move into the region and "forestall any sectarian agency from getting control."[101]

Victoria's Salvation Army Matson Lodge, opened in 1955, is an excellent illustration of the new ideas in institutional architecture for old age homes. The west coast firm of Wade, Stockdill and Armour provided plans for a new building with a view across Victoria Harbour to the Olympic Mountains beyond. The "guest rooms," as they were called in a 1962 *Royal Architectural Institute of Canada Journal* article, radiated out in two directions from a central hub corridor that contained the dining room, the lounge, a shop, a library, a television room, and a radio room. The centrality of these communal rooms in the overall design indicates a new emphasis on sociability. The circular lounge, with its sweeping panoramic views and tasteful modern furniture and houseplants, was a particular feature of the design, and one appreciated by the residents. The accoutrements were of a middle-class home, although the scale was clearly institutional. Overall, the emphasis within the building's design was away from the external community, toward either the magnificent view or the internal world of the old age home with its wide range of services for residents. The sweeping

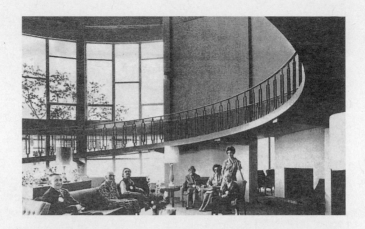

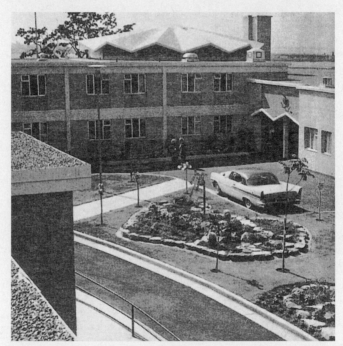

Interior and exterior views of the Salvation Army's Matson Lodge, Victoria, 1950s. These views of this philanthropic facility, designed by the architectural firm of Wade, Stockdill and Armour in the early 1950s, demonstrate both the new emphasis on middle-class sociability within the old age home and the shift away from interaction with the outside community, inward toward the world of the old age home with its stunning vista from the lounge. (National Library, Ottawa)

Y-shaped driveway up to the building, with large central flower beds, appears to have been designed with vehicle rather than pedestrian traffic in mind.[102]

There was a similar expansion of ethnic old age homes, all located in Vancouver and run by Scandinavian groups. In 1944 the Western Canadian Danish Society built a home for twenty-four elderly Danish-Canadians in rural Burnaby; a decade later there was accommodation for forty men and women at Dania.[103] In 1947 the Icelandic community converted a large former guest house in the affluent Shaunnessy district into Icelandic Home, a residence for thirty elderly Icelandic-Canadian citizens. The ground floor had a spacious drawing room, matron's quarters, kitchen, and dining room. There were three other levels to the facility, with rooms for one, two, or three people and two further rooms in the basement. The *Canadian Welfare* article that lauded the efforts of the Danish and Icelandic communities for their elderly also reported the construction of a residence for fifty elderly Swedish-Canadians in North Vancouver.[104]

While private institutions did not match charitable or municipal facilities in innovative design, they were vigorous in terms of growth in patient numbers. Throughout the 1940s and 1950s, smaller facilities closed and were replaced by larger enterprises. This growth indicates that a small private hospital for the aged was no longer a viable business for a single woman. Provincial bureaucrats and policy-makers were anxious to curb the size and power of private hospitals, but small operators were sometimes unable to provide the level of facilities and service that provincial hospital inspectors now saw as mandatory for aged men and women. Moreover, as was the case in other economic sectors, corporate interests were attracted to the business of providing care for the elderly by the new economic opportunity presented by government financing for individual patients and by rising public demand.[105]

A look at private hospitals in Victoria and the adjoining municipalities of Oak Bay, Saanich, and Esquimalt demonstrates how this pattern evolved. Throughout the 1930s there were approximately eight private hospitals providing care for the chronically ill and convalescent in the area. As was the case earlier, this was a women's business and small enterprise. Of the hospitals listed at this time, only the Menzies Nursing Home was licensed to someone other than the superintendent directly responsible for the daily administration of the facility. The Menzies establishment was also the only private hospital whose license was not held by a woman. The number of beds in the Victoria institutions ranged from five to nineteen, with the three largest institutions being those that took municipal cases. By 1950 seven of these small private hospitals, some of which had been operating since the 1920s, had closed their doors. The Menzies Nursing Home, control of which had been transferred to Miss Kathleen Dann, the superintendent, became a welfare institution in 1948.[106]

New enterprises with greater capital for expansion began to take over. In 1951 Mrs and Mr Boel opened a twelve-bed private hospital on Rockland Avenue, not far from the Caroline Macklem Home. They added six beds to the establishment in 1954, and sold the business to another couple in 1958. Miss Jane Nixon, manager of the Saanich Health Centre (Royal Oak Private Hospital) since 1940, turned her license over to Mr and Mrs Emery in 1952. Owned by a limited company, Clovelly Private Hospital in Saanich began operating in 1949 with twenty-six beds. By 1951 the hospital had thirty patients in the main building and a two-room cottage where the charge nurse lived. In 1958 the hospital added another twelve beds to make a total of forty-two.[107]

Clear codes of practice and provision for private hospitals in B.C. had evolved by the mid-1950s. The provincial inspector of hospitals determined official bed capacity at 80 square feet of floor space per patient in a room shared with two or more other people, 100 square feet of floor space per patient in a semi-private room, and 120 square feet of floor space in a private room. Bathroom facilities were required on all floors used by patients. A nurse's station and controlled supply cupboard for medications was not only required but also had to be shown on proposed floor plans for new facilities. Each patient bed was to be equipped with a call bell for the nurse and an individual light. There were also strict fire regulations and standards for the width of halls and doorways to allow free movement of beds.[108]

While independent women were no longer operating small private hospitals, women provided the majority of boarding home care for elderly public charges. Indeed, women who had trouble meeting higher standards for private hospitals may have been shifting downward in the care hierarchy, seeking licenses to provide boarding home care. Olive Clark, for example, gave up her private hospital licence in 1946 but subsequently applied for permission to give "care, food and lodging to four aged persons" in her Saanich home.[109] In the late 1940s, the municipality of Saanich also boarded elderly men unable to live alone but not in need of extensive nursing care at Miss Nixon's boarding home on Gorge Road or with Edith Smith in her Logan Avenue home. These were very small operations: Nixon took in eight old people and Smith had room for six.[110]

Women such as Olive Clark and Edith Smith began taking small numbers of hospital clearance cases into their homes in the 1930s and

1940s, and this trend continued in the post-war period. As these cases suggest, registered boarding homes for elderly men and women were usually small, with only three to one dozen residents, and were often operated by married women. Boarding homes for aged ex-hospital patients usually matched the size of the community in which they were situated. Mrs Sarah Fox of Kelowna had four or five old people boarding in her home during the 1940s. In 1944 Mrs E.A. Robinson of the small settlement of Enderby took in two elderly boarders.[111]

Vancouver's larger population base meant that there were many more registered boarding homes for old people – a total of 490 in 1949 – than in smaller urban centres, and that these facilities were also larger and run on professional lines.[112] Mayfair Home, for instance, had fifty-two residents and operated under the administration of a matron. Among the Vancouver boarding houses tabulated in the late 1940s, approximately two-thirds of the residents were men. One commercial boarding house for men, located near the junction of Broadway and Granville streets and surveyed in 1948, was an old house with single and double rooms. Each resident had a closet, a bed, an easy chair, and a dresser. There was no communal sitting or dining room.[113]

Many small boarding homes operated for less than a year, and guests and hosts often shared living space in the family home. Olive Thomas, who applied to the Corporation of Saanich for permission to operate a boarding home in 1947, proposed to accommodate three elderly people in rooms on the main floor of her family house. The authorities acknowledged that the rooms would be noisy with four young children in the house, but added "this would constitute only a minor objection."[114] In 1939, Mrs Meyer of Revelstoke offered a home to an old man in the two-story white frame house where she lived with her husband.[115]

Registered boarding homes in Vancouver, like their sister institutions in Victoria and elsewhere, served as "half-way houses" to nursing homes, providing custodial care for those who could not manage on their own but did not require nursing attention.[116] Like most institutional accommodation for the elderly before the mid-1950s, licensed boarding homes in Vancouver were usually converted family dwellings. Many of these older buildings had pleasing features like oak panelling, bay windows, gracious entrance halls, and large verandas: one residence for retired women had "sheer frilly white curtains at the windows and sealers of home-made jam in the kitchen." A 1948 observer noted comfortable chairs, good lighting, and a well-equipped kitchen. But these borrowed buildings clearly had functional limitations as institutions for the aged. Only two of the facilities considered in the 1948 survey had communal dining and sitting rooms. In one home for women, fifteen residents and the matron shared a single bathroom. In another seventeen women shared one full bathroom and a separate toilet while the twenty male residents had the use of two full bathrooms. The sleeping quarters in these boarding homes varied: there were some private rooms, while in other cases as many as six men shared a larger dormitory.[117]

As was the case with municipal old age homes, the 1940s and 1950s were a period of considerable growth in charitable and private accommodation for B.C.'s elderly. Supported by provincial funds, religious and ethnic groups converted older dwellings and established new purpose-built homes for old people. The design of new facilities showed a growing interest in the aged as a unique social group. Private hospitals and boarding homes for elderly public clients also flourished, evolving from small operations run by women to larger establishments owned by corporations or families.

Institutional care for the elderly in British Columbia began in the late nineteenth century with a handful of public and charitable institutions. These first facilities were meant to reward men and women who had contributed to the founding of a new province. Poorhouse codes inevitably found expression in the architecture and administration of these institutions, but they were not founded as workhouses as were the facilities used for the indigent aged in central and eastern Canada. State and charitable old age homes remained scarce until nearly midway through the twentieth century.

At the close of the Second World War, with the elderly occupying a recognized place on the post-war social agenda and the assurance of funding from public patients and provincial building funds, the number of municipal and philanthropic old age homes increased dramatically. For the first time, the old age home was designed with a specific clientele of elderly people in mind. Architecturally, this new old age home was stamped with the cultural ethos of middle-class Canada. In the organization of space in both old and new facilities, the old age home was becoming a medical facility rather than a welfare institution.

Public and private hospitals were also used to house elderly men and women too frail or too poor to live independently. Over time, the use of general hospitals for this group of old people would prove to be problematic. The use of private hospitals for the indigent elderly, however, was a more enduring pattern, and by the 1940s private hospitals caring for the aged had increased dramatically both in size and in number.[118]

Overall, this history of institutional development speaks most directly to the low status of the aged on the policy agenda. New institutions are costly ventures. Apart from the first flush of institutional enthusiasm in the late nineteenth and early twentieth centuries, homes for the elderly were secondhand facilities. Between 1915 and 1951, with the exception of Mount Saint Mary's, no new public old age homes were built in B.C. After the Second World War, with the elderly indigent rehabilitated as the "senior citizen," homes for the aged regained their earlier status as monuments to a compassionate society and the pioneering efforts of the men and women who had spent their youth building the province.

3 The Old Age Home Revisioned: The Nursing Home Ideal

Pushed by public pressure and new professional concerns, efforts were made throughout the 1940s and 1950s to sever the historical link between the workhouse and the old age home and to reshape residential accommodation for the aged into middle-class medical institutions. The growth of interest in old age and concerns about institutional provision for the infirm and indigent elderly followed a similar pattern in Canada, the United States, Britain, and Australia.[1] Public geriatric institutions were scorned for being too regimented, for having a "prison-like atmosphere," and for being irrelevant reminders of the antiquated Poor Law in the modern welfare state.[2] H.S. Farquhar, Nova Scotia's director of old age pensions, expressed the general opinion of professionals in a 1946 statement: "In many parts of our land, we find almost unchanged the old poor house where the aged are housed with the senile and sick. Endless idle days, dull monotony until death comes as a welcome release."[3] Many believed that highly structured institutions with a punitive attitude toward their residents actually undermined the health of the aged men and women who lived there.[4]

These ideas were common currency in British Columbia both among health and social welfare professionals and in the larger public community. But what was to replace the poorhouse? The professional agenda was most clearly outlined in the western province by Isobel Harvey, a provincial bureaucrat and social worker, in her 1945 "Study of Chronic Disease in British Columbia." Harvey's institutional ideal brought together elements of modern medical practice, rehabilitative therapy, welfare professionalism, compassionate care for the aged, and the middle-class family home. Staff should be kind and understanding to their aged patients, but always professionally trained. Space and resources should be allocated for physiotherapy and occupational therapy, yet a "homelike atmosphere" was also of paramount importance. If care was not taken to implement new ideas concerning the institutionalized elderly, Harvey warned, "there is a grave danger of something like the old 'poor farm' rearing its ugly head in British Columbia."[5]

A series of 1947 Vancouver newspaper editorials about the Marpole (earlier the Home for Incurables) and Allco branches of the Provincial Infirmary brought together the main elements of public criticism and demonstrated a convergence between lay and professional opinion. "That Place at Marpole," the argument held, was overcrowded, unsafe, and lacking modern medical equipment, recreational facilities, and professional input from a psychiatrist or a nutritionist. Moreover, its inner-city location, at "a particularly busy and noisy tram and highway intersection," jarred with the perceived idea of what a home for the aged should be. The close of life should come in a cheerful, peaceful place, where patients lived and died in comfort. Shifting the focus to Allco, the *Vancouver Province* cited a dearth of nurses or doctors resident at the facility and the lack of occupational therapy and physiotherapy programs that left the residents with nothing to do. "Marpole and Allco," one writer concluded, "are anachronisms. They do not belong to this age or this province."[6]

These criticisms were manifestations of wider social, political, and professional shifts. The state, health and social welfare professionals, and the public community now shared a new commitment to a compassionate society where those in need would be cared for in comfort. A residential facility for elderly public patients was no longer to be a punishment for a life of irresponsibility but a respectable "home" for worthy citizens in their old age. An awareness of growing numbers of elderly people in the general population, and of the challenges posed by this demographic shift, was met by the beginnings of gerontological specialization. Health and social welfare professionals made the old age home part of their professional terrain, redefining inmates as patients in need of their expert attention. The ideological force of the middle class as a measuring stick for normality also made its mark on the old age home: facilities were meant to be modelled on something midway between the post-war suburban family home and the modern hospital. A new belief in recreation as a route to physical and mental well-being, another facet of middle-class culture and post-war social policy, also left its mark on institutions for the elderly. In the context of the old age home, then, modernity meant professionalism and compassion amidst middle-class comforts and surroundings.

However, while the immediate post-war period was a time of optimism and a renewed belief in the power of the professional state to build a healthier and more egalitarian society, even in the 1940s strong cultural forces within Canadian society made revolutionary changes to the old age home impossible. I have already described in chapter 2 the post-war difficulty of finding supplies and labour to build new old age homes, but the problem was more than just logistics. A great block to change was the ageism inherent within professional responses to elderly people. Moreover, the professional groups who became most closely connected with the old age home were largely female and therefore lacked the power of male-dominated professional sectors. So old age homes remained second-rate on two counts.

This chapter looks at different facets of the new agenda for old age homes. I begin with the professional colonization of the old age home and the recreation of "inmates" into "patients." The next section deals with the outward trappings of the reformed old age home, discussing ways in which new names and a new décor moved the institution closer to a middle-class, medical model. I then consider how wider societal concerns about chronic illness and physical fitness were grafted onto the agenda of the new institution. The last section explores elements of professional ageism and the creation of a new "ideal" resident for the old age home, an image often at odds with the men and women who actually lived in these places.

PROFESSIONALS IN THE OLD AGE HOME

Health and social welfare professionals were pivotal players in the transformation of the poorhouse to the old age home. The growth of their power was both structural and ideological, with the Marpole branch of the Provincial Infirmary system acting as a flagship institution for change in B.C.[7] Administrative procedures adopted by the infirmary system in 1938 empowered doctors and social workers to act as the new gatekeepers to public old age homes in the province, replacing the provincial policemen, government agents, and relief workers. Inside the institution the work of core staff was now supplemented by a range of specialists that included social workers, occupational thaerapists, physiotherapists, and nutritionists.

The process of professional colonization was a part of a broader interest in old people that emerged in the inter-war years. British and American sociologists, physicians, and scientists began actively building the foundations of modern gerontology during the first decades of the twentieth century,[8] but Canadian interest in the emerging speciality did not come until the final years of the Depression.[9] From that point there was a steady increase in the number of articles on old age published in Canadian medical and social work journals. Professional and governmental groups were set up to study aging.[10] By the end of the Second World War Canadian doctors, social workers, and bureaucrats saw the aged as a vulnerable group with specific social and medical problems.

B.C. fit well into this national and continental professional paradigm. The Committee on the Care of the Aged, a sub-committee of the Family Division of Greater Vancouver, began meeting in 1943. Between 1948 and 1960 seventeen University of British Columbia social work students completed master's theses on old age. The question of institutional care for the elderly was an area of particular interest, and health and social welfare professionals established themselves as experts in this regard. In an institutional setting, they maintained, aged men and women required their special skills,[11] and doctors, nurses, social workers, physiotherapists, and occupational therapists came to regard the elderly and old age homes as part of their jurisdiction. They now had the power to make judgments concerning the diagnosis and treatment of elderly residents, a kind of cultural control that superintendents and staff of older poor law institutions had never had. Professional authority became built into both the culture and the administrative structure of the old age home.[12] Overall, social workers and nurses, rather than physcans, dominated professional discussion about old age and homes for the elderly at this time.

The Provincial Infirmary at the Marpole branch illustrates the importance of administrative reform and professional input in the reconceptualized old age home: the custodial institution became a medical facility. The transformation of Marpole began in 1938, just as the broader academic and professional interest in gerontology was developing. Visiting the facility, Assistant Provincial Health Officer Gregoire Amyot and Provincial Inspector of Hospitals Percy Ward made a number of recommendations designed to bring conditions at Marpole in line with broader health and welfare reforms in the province.[13]

A new focus on the study and treatment of Marpole residents and the creation of professional institutional hierarchies were key recommendations of the 1938 study. Professional input into the institution increased in a number of ways. An Infirmary Advisory Board of departmental officials and "experts" was appointed in February 1938 to meet on a regular basis to discuss administrative problems and policy directions. Institutional administrators were encouraged to make use of the range of specialist services, including the mental health, tuberculosis, venereal disease divisions, the laboratory, and the Welfare Field Service.[14]

Figure 1
Poorhouse "ideal inmate" vs nursing home
"ideal patient"

"Ideal inmate"

- hard-working
- obedient
- does not make trouble with other inmates

"Ideal patient"

- participates in therapy
- well-behaved
- social/part of the institutional "family"

The dual positions of matron and medical superintendent, which had caused conflict in leadership within the Home, were replaced by a single superintendent directly responsible to the deputy provincial secretary.[15] As figure 1 illustrates, doctors and social workers took over from relief officers and government agents as the gatekeepers of public facilities for the elderly, and thereby transformed the task of gatekeeping from a purely administrative function to a pyscho-medical exercise.[16]

Under the guidance of "expert" staff, Marpole was to be run on a medical model, with regularized procedures that would chart the physical and mental health of each patient. Dr West was appointed visiting physician to the Provincial Infirmary and a medical survey of all patients was undertaken. A system of detailed medical and social patient records was created and physical examinations of residents became routine. Incoming residents were given a thorough physical examination by a physician, and the 1943 annual report of the institution noted that all residents were being given a blood test upon admission. A decade later all incoming patients were sent for medical screening to either the Vancouver General Hospital or St Joseph's Hospital in Victoria: "The organized medical staff of these two institutions diagnose each case; advise on treatments; set out prognosis and generally assist the attending physician at each branch."[17]

Medical supervision of the institutionalized elderly became the accepted standard, and its absence was commented upon. The 1949 annual report of the Welfare Institutions Licensing Board noted that the majority of state-licensed boarding homes now had a regular attending physician.[18] In a 1944 article for *Canadian Welfare,* Laura Holland, then adviser on social policy for the provincial government, held up the Soroptimist House in Vancouver as a model, with its resident matron to provide medical supervision for the older women who lived there.[19]

A parallel process took place at Marpole in the field of social work. Following the 1938 survey, Zella M. Collins, a senior social worker and administrator with the provincial Welfare Field Service, was assigned to create a system of numerical files and patient case histories for the institution. Collins placed her own professional stamp on admittance procedures at the Provincial Infirmary: henceforth, every application was to be accompanied by a social history of the individual. Workers from the Welfare Field Service became adjunct workers for the infirmary system, funnelling appropriate patients into the institution accompanied by well-documented case files.[20]

The use of social casework techniques and routine medical examinations meant that medical and social work professionals now had a much more intimate knowledge of the institutionalized elderly in their care. The body and the life story became part of the professional mapping of the elderly resident: the aged man or woman under scrutiny was now professional property. A 1943 memo written by Percy Ward stressed the importance of social work in dealing with infirmary residents: "To make satisfactory placements we must bring all relatives and interested parties into consideration and we must know all about these people, if we are to use good judgement in caring for the clients."[21] Individual cases and situations were now defined by medical and social work ideas about appropriate behaviour, care, and treatment of the aged.

With a new focus on the elderly as a unique category of clients, a notion of specialized institutional care for older women and men took shape. This new way of ordering institutional care was evident in the hierarchy of geriatric institutions that had evolved in B.C. by the late 1940s: boarding homes, private hospitals, and public hospitals for the chronically ill.[22] Professionals and administrators argued that the elderly should now be professionally assessed to gauge their physical and mental health and placed in an appropriate institution. A 1957 document, sent by F. Heaton, an administrator for the municipality of Saanich, to Donald Cox, deputy minister of Hospital Insurance, shows how systems of classification evolved. Heaton divided the elderly into four categories: the healthy, the infirm, the sick, and the psychiatric. With ongoing evaluation and therapeutic help, old people might move from one category to another. Residential accommodation was, of course, to be chosen in accordance with classification. Heaton recommended the establishment of geriatric assessment and research departments in general hospitals to stream elderly people into the correct institution.[23]

Professional interest grew in cataloguing the intimacies of the bodies, minds, and personal histories of institutionalized old people. By the early 1960s Dr Doris Mackay, a specialist in rehabilitative medicine, was able to subdivide patients in private hospitals into six categories, based on the level of care that they required. Reviewing patient populations at thirteen facilities in Greater Vancouver and Victoria, Mackay gathered information on a set of criteria that ranged from financial solvency to bowel and bladder continence. The mental state of patients was also evaluated. Although Mackay's data provided strong evidence of patient improvement through wider use of occupational therapy and physiotherapy, she cautioned against placing patients from different classifications alongside one another in old age homes.[24]

Extra-institutional input into the daily routine of old age homes also became more professionalized with the growing involvement of occupational therapists, physiotherapists, and, ultimately, nutritionists (see figure 1). Occupational therapy was the first new professional enterprise to enter the old age home. Work, considered a form of therapy for mental health patients, had never been presented as more than standard poor law practice at the Provincial Home for Old Men or the Old People's Home in Vancouver. Occupational therapists working in old age homes transformed poor law labour into a therapeutic experience, creating an entirely new field of expertise.

Again, the most dynamic institution in terms of occupational therapy and physiotherapy was the Provincial Infirmary at Marpole. Somewhat ironically, the initial involvement of this group of extra-institutional practitioners owed their professional place inside the old age home to the crusading efforts of the voluntary Women's Auxiliary. Faced with bureaucratic intransigence, the powerful auxiliary went over the heads of provincial administrators to hire the first part-time occupational therapist in the late 1930s. In this sense the Women's Auxiliary, highly organized and willing to use their power to push professionals into place at Marpole, was a very different kind of extra-institutional group than the charity workers who took Christmas fare to the Old Men's Home in Victoria. The Marpole Women's Auxiliary was clearly a pressure group, not professionals themselves but connected to the world of professionals by marriage and class alliances. By 1944 an occupational therapy program had been formally established at the Allco and Marpole branches of the Provincial Infirmary.[25]

The story of physiotherapy is similar. Geriatric physiotherapy had begun in England during the 1930s with the development of exercise programs to increase the activity of stroke patients.[26] Interest in this field soon spread to Canada. Two years after the occupational therapy program had set down roots, a part-time physiotherapist was added to the Marpole staff. Although there was less enthusiasm for such therapeutics among the Sisters of Saint Ann, who ran Mount Saint Mary's in Victoria, the 1946 report of the Provincial Infirmary noted that a part-time physiotherapist had joined their staff.[27]

Nutritionists became involved in old age homes during the 1940s as well. By 1942 Superintendent Motherwell was lobbying for a separate "diet kitchen" at Marpole.[28] M. Baldwin, nutritional consultant with the provincial Board of Health, visited the Provincial Home in 1945. Her report shows how Canada's Food Rules were applied to a clientele of institutionalized elderly people. Arguing that well-balanced meals were essential to the quality of life in old age, Baldwin recommended the use of seasonings and tasty appetizers to encourage reluctant eaters and advised against heavy meals at noon and full-fat milk, which would encourage constipation among the old men. "Our aim in the care of the aged," Baldwin concluded, "is to 'Add life to years rather than years to life.'"[29]

Women dominated the ranks of the new professionals now finding employment within the walls of the old age home, as social workers, nutritionists, physiotherapists, and occupational therapists.[30] Outside of social work, I found no men hired as professionals for these positions during the period studied. With their special nurturing qualities and their cultural connection with "the home," women were seen as essential in a modern compassionate institution for the aged. Both professionals and government bureaucrats looked for maternal qualities in caregivers, implicitly suggesting that women were most suitable for aged patients.[31]

This maternalism had all the heavy-handed properties of traditional paternalism. Professional writing repeatedly stressed the "female" or "maternal" qualities of professionals in the old age home. An equation of the elderly with children is evident. The best kind of social worker or nurse, these authors maintained, was someone who would be sympathetic and understanding, make sure that their elderly patients or clients were dressed in appropriate clothing, and encourage interests and hobbies. A 1947 article in *Canadian Nurse* told its readers that old people "are forgetful, tend to reminisce and to fabricate. Therefore, the nurse caring for these people should be kind, understanding, and willing to take time to listen sympathetically to their stories."[32] Social workers were to act as intermediaries, taking on the female role as peacemaker to smooth over differences between patients, families, administrators, staff, and doctors.[33]

In her 1942 annual report, Marpole superintendent Motherwell proudly stated that "[t]he treatment of the aged is now being recognised as a special branch of Medicine."[34] This was a profound, if well-intentioned, overstatement. Mainstream medicine remained uninterested in the old and their illnesses. Innovative surgical techniques and medical technology could not yet be used for this group of patients. The absence of men from professional ranks within the old age home

was another indication of the secondary status of these facilities and
the ageist equation of the elderly with children.

But viewed from a broader professional perspective, B.C.'s old age
homes of the 1940s were an excellent forum for professional colonization. The Provincial Infirmary at Marpole was the flagship institution in this regard, but expectations and aspirations were spread much
more widely at the end of the decade. By 1950 a "good" old age home
was increasingly seen as one that was staffed by medical and social
welfare professionals and run along regularized administrative lines. It
would also have staff and facilities for occupational therapy and physiotherapy. In the professional mind, residents were transformed from
poor law inmates into social work clients and medical patients. The
dominance of women among institutional and extra-institutional staff,
both as professionals and non-professionals, reflected the strong social
belief that women were vital nurturers and "homemakers."

DISCARDING THE POORHOUSE –
CREATING THE OLD AGE HOME

B.C.'s health and welfare professionals worked hard to leave the poorhouse behind. Part of this process was cosmetic, refashioning the
public face of residential accommodation for the elderly and recreating
the interior of such facilities to resemble respectable "homes" rather
than harsh institutions. As Elaine Tyler May makes clear in her work
on the American family during the Cold War era, the external and
internal organization and appearance of family dwellings was an
important characteristic of post-war society.[35] The same held true for
old age homes. The goal was to extinguish the image of the old age
home as a punitive place of last resort, the tall, gloomy workhouse of
Dickensian mythology. The reformed old age home would be fit for
the newly minted "senior citizen."[36] It would be a modern, single-story
complex, decorated inside with light paint rather than dark stained
wood. Communal areas would bring together residents for social
events rather than merely for meals. This suggests a middle-class family
home, but there were allusions to the medical functions of the buildings as well.

With limited funds and supplies for building new old age homes,
names were at first the strongest public statement of this institutional
rebirth.[37] From the late 1930s there was a distinct shift in the names
bestowed on old age homes and many older institutions were renamed.
Donald W. Cox, commissioner of the British Columbia Hospital Insurance Service, stated in a 1948 conference presentation that "[o]ne
significant indication of late is the sweeping away of the old inhuman

titles such as 'Home for Incurables,' which frequently destroy the last vestige of hope in the patient; and the substitution of hospital names that in no way 'label' the hospital or the patient."[38] Institutional names discarded through the late 1930s and 1940s in B.C. included the Provincial Home for Incurables, the Home for Aged and Infirm Ladies, the Old People's Home (Vancouver), and the Old Men's Home (Victoria). The only public old age home in the province that retained its original title was the Provincial Home for Old Men in Kamloops.

As Cox's presentation suggests, administrators chose names that obscured the charitable or poor law functions and history of these facilities. There were several new trends in titles for old age homes, patterns that were also followed in Ontario during the same period.[39] Some institutions were given titles that evoked a curative, healing image, a quiet place for the last stage of life. Other new names alluded to a hospital or a gracious family home. The Home for Incurables became the Provincial Infirmary in 1937 – the first public institution in the province to undergo this public transformation. Similarly, the names of new facilities such as the Victoria Nursing Home, renamed the Gorge Road Hospital in 1954, reflected the hope that homes for the aged could serve to rehabilitate, or actually cure, elderly men and women.

A second post-war trend was to name an institution after a worthy public figure, indicating both the growing respectability of old age homes and an aspiration for higher status in the public community. Thus, Vancouver's Old People's Home was renamed Taylor Manor in 1947, honouring a former mayor of the city. The new title was part of a broader set of institutional reforms designed to make the facility more appealing to Vancouver's elderly.[40] In Kelowna, the new municipal home was named after a popular local politician.

A third pattern were names that presented the old age home as a place for recreation. In 1950 the Home for Aged and Infirm Ladies in Victoria was transformed into Rose Manor, a reference to the beautiful gardens surrounding the building. The new name might also have been an allusion to an English country home, a not uncommon custom in Victoria, one of B.C.'s most "English" communities. When the Oliver and District Senior Citizen's Society opened an old age home in 1957, the new facility was called "Sunnybank" after a favoured English location.

Victoria's Old Men's Home was listed in the 1952 city directory as Mountain View, a name suggesting a contemplative vista on the last stage of life.[41] It was not widely used, however: city officials and the public held fast to the older title. This may have been because of the similarity between the new name and Valleyview and Skeenaview, two new psychiatric facilities for B.C.'s elderly mental health patients established during the period. Names with what Peter Townsend called "a faint echo of gloomy foreboding" were also used, such as Eventide for the municipal home in Prince Rupert.[42]

Home was of course a powerful theme in the years following the disruption of the Second World War, when families had to work so hard to find places to live,[43] and it occurs frequently in the literature calling for institutional rebirth. Social work student Dennis Guest detailed efforts to reshape an unpopular institution into a respectable home for the aged in his 1952 study of Vancouver's Taylor Manor. In 1945 city officials redefined it as a "home" rather than a public poorhouse. Guest described the process, placing particular emphasis on the word "home": "The most difficult task was trying to remove the stigma of an institution that had, during the depression, filled the role of that most odious of all institutions, the workhouse. Related to this was the job of converting the Old People's Home from an institution into a place that could really be called a *home* for the aged."[44]

The notion of creating a "home" out of an institution was most clearly expressed in interior decoration. The author of a 1944 report detailing the need for a new old age home in Victoria stressed the importance of a "cheerful and homelike" environment, arguing that this kind of atmosphere was in itself therapeutic.[45] In fact, in long-established facilities, interior décor became even more critical in the drive to banish the image of the poorhouse. Redecorating schemes, it was felt, "modernized" old buildings, putting further distance between the poor law purpose for which the institution had been intended and the revisioned nursing home.

Like Dennis Guest, Isobel Harvey stressed the importance of turning the institution into a "home" when she surveyed the Kamloops Provincial Home in 1945. Harvey suggested that a "beautifully constructed room," presently unused, could be made into "the centre of the Home." All that was needed, she argued, was the addition of comfortable chairs, reading lamps, drapes, and games tables, items typical of the middle-class family home. In Harvey's vision, these decorative changes would draw inmates out from their individual bedrooms and make the institution a happier place.[46]

Redecoration schemes were also underway at the Marpole branch of the Provincial Infirmary in the early 1940s. The auditorium, evidently the social nexus for the institution's patients, was transformed with new curtains, standard lamps, easy chairs, and sofas. "New red tops with monometal trimmings" were fixed onto the first floor tables. The fact that the institution's enthusiastic Women's Auxiliary had been responsible for donating all the new furnishings except for the drapes suggests that women, particularly middle-class volunteers, were key agents of this process.[47] The minute books of Rose Manor indicate that a similar process was underway at charitable homes. Although the Home Committee always took a considerable interest in new linen, furnishings, and wall coverings, the 1952 annual report noted that "[m]any improvements have been made throughout the Home during the year – rooms and corridors painted, new linoleum laid, new drapes and covers added where necessary, all adding to the comforts of home surroundings."[48]

In passages describing this transformation images of colour and light are juxtaposed against the drabness and darkness of the past. There is an obvious parallel to what was taking place at the same time in Ontario, and to Olive Matthew's British campaign to "bring more colour into the lives of old people in institutions," although there is no indication that Harvey and her colleagues were drawing directly on ideas from these places.[49] At the Vancouver Old People's Home woodwork and walls were painted in lighter colours.[50] At the Kamloops institution dark woodwork and drab colours were covered by plywood panelling and white paint. Grey blankets were replaced by rose-coloured throws on Marpole's women's wards. The installation of personal bedside lights was a feature of the period. Small bed lamps were donated by the Marpole Women's Auxiliary in 1941, and three years later extra electrical outlets were put in all the sleeping quarters to bring more light into the rooms.[51] Floor to ceiling windows and large modern table lamps dominated the circular lounge at the Salvation Army's Matson Lodge in Victoria.[52]

What was the deeper message behind the semiotics of renaming and redecorating the old age home? Names and beauty are never inconsequential, but ultimately these cosmetic changes only facilitated a public and professional denial about institutions for the elderly. Although many people probably appreciated a chance to grab a comfortable chair in a freshly painted sitting room, redecorating and renaming institutions were really cinematic devices to draw the viewer's attention away from the smoking gun. "Home" is meant to be a place where you chose to live with people you love. Old age homes are institutions where people live in the last stage of life and, often, where they die, shut off from family and friends. New names and new paint might obscure this reality, but they could not alter it.

There is a strong statement about class and care here as well. Residential facilities for the elderly were no longer to be places of last resort for impoverished old men on society's margins. Instead, residents drawn from across a broad social spectrum would receive professional care in a homelike setting. These were to be kinder places, where residents would be treated in a more egalitarian fashion, living integrated lives in well-decorated surroundings. But this new ideal facility was not classless. The notion of institutions as "homes" drew upon the culture of the middle-class family, a place where many of the professionals working in the old age home had begun their lives, but the majority of their patients had not.

CHRONIC ILLNESS, OCCUPATIONAL THERAPY, AND RECREATION

Broader health concerns about the rise of chronic illness and the need for a fit populace also shaped the professional agenda for old age homes in the 1940s and 1950s. Health care professionals believed that the rise in chronic disease was due to the increasing number of men and women who lived to old age and became chronically ill in their last decades. If these people could be treated and released from hospital, then public money could be saved and much needed hospital beds secured. Moreover, if chronic illness was treatable, then some aspects of the aging process could also be eradicated.[53]

Reflecting the wider social preoccupation with recreation in the post-war period, recreational activity came to be regarded as the key to a healthy old age. In the activity model of aging, which became an inherent part of professional attitudes toward the elderly, planned activities were to take the place of work in the lives of retired people. This ideological position fit well with the post-war middle-class myth of retirement as a "golden age." Hobbies, exercise, or participation in a community seniors club were advocated as routes to full citizenship and positive living.[54] Community-based recreational programs for seniors were created during the late 1940s at Gordon House in Vancouver's west end and in New Westminster, Port Alberni, Kamloops, and Kelowna.[55]

This belief in the curative powers of recreation in old age extended to homes for the elderly. Throughout the 1940s government administrators argued for medically supervised recreational programs in state and commercial facilities, stating that the healthy aged were cheaper to maintain in an institution than the frail and sickly.[56] Laura Holland, the prominent B.C. social worker and bureaucrat mentioned earlier, believed that the taxpayer would benefit from medically supervised recreational programs run by the state in licensed boarding homes. Writing in 1941, Holland argued that such policy would delay many conditions of senility that, when they reached the "public nuisance" stage, necessitated admission to a mental hospital or some other form of custodial care or supervision.[57]

Old age homes, chronic illness, and recreation became closely linked in the minds of professionals and government bureaucrats involved with B.C.'s old age homes. A growing awareness of the high cost of caring for the chronically ill was coupled with a rising belief in the curative potential of rehabilitative medicine. Health professionals and bureaucrats thought that some of the illnesses of old age could be successfully treated in an institutional setting. Moreover, if aged men and women could be provided with health care that would ensure that they remained fit, then institutionalization might be delayed or avoided. Edith Pringle, provincial inspector of hospitals, argued in 1953 that, "[g]iven proper care, these ailments (diseases common to old age) can, in some cases, be prevented. In others, they may be postponed, and, in still others, life can be more enjoyable and productive."[58]

There was much discussion, particularly in the immediate post-war period, concerning the need for a purpose-built chronic disease hospital in B.C., perhaps forming a wing of a general hospital or situated apart from the city in a tranquil setting.[59] Such a facility, it was believed, would free general hospitals to deal with those with acute conditions. It was acknowledged that old people would comprise the majority of the clientele. But without the political will to fund a new chronic hospital, the Provincial Infirmary at Marpole became the nucleus of professional initiatives in the treatment of chronic illness in B.C. Programs begun by occupational therapists and physiotherapists and volunteers at the Vancouver facility became the model for institutions across the province.

Government reports lauded occupational therapy and physiotherapy efforts at Marpole and repeatedly criticized Mount Saint Mary's for failing to provide adequate occupational therapy programs for their patients. The Marpole occupational therapy department quickly became a positive note in the infirmary superintendent's annual reports and a point of praise in surveys of the Provincial Infirmary system. In 1945 the institution's annual report noted that the Hon. W.C. Woodward, lieutenant governor of British Columbia, had shown a special interest in the occupational therapy department during his June visit to the institution. The 1950 Provincial Infirmaries Report stated that "Occupational Therapy continues, more patients are interested in handicrafts, a new Occupational Therapy studio with wide sun decks is being built, there is public interest in this department and the Women's Auxiliary take a strong role."[60]

The new Victoria Nursing Home (later the Gorge Road Hospital) fit well into new ideas concerning the value of occupational therapy and physiotherapy for the aged and chronically ill. From the institution's beginning in 1944 the goal of rehabilitating patients through the use of occupational therapy was clearly articulated. The institution expanded significantly in patient numbers during the period.[61]

The 1949 report of the Welfare Institutions Licensing Board noted that "all homes for old people are being encouraged to pay more attention to the recreational and occupational needs of the guests."[62]

This concept of recreation was different from the picnics, outings, and entertainment that had been characteristic fare at the Vancouver Old People's Home and the Victoria Old Men's Home in the early twentieth century. The recreation being prescribed by Laura Holland and Isobel Harvey stressed physical activity and group participation. Sociologists of the period believed that group work served an array of purposes: it met the emotional needs of the individual, encouraged learning, and discouraged anti-social behaviour.[63] Administrators of old age homes in B.C. were open to these ideas, although public institutions were generally more quick to adopt new professional practices. As the superintendent of the Provincial Home stated in 1955, "participation, in any manner whatsoever, is the best therapy."[64]

At the Kamloops facility inmates were encouraged to take daily walks, feed the birds, work in the garden or on the farm, attend sporting events, and play pool. Administrators at Marpole built up the library and bought three new radios and fifty earphones so that patients could keep pace with the world outside the institution. After the Second World War administrators at the Vancouver Old People's Home installed a radio in the common room and put a putting green in the grounds. The 1950–51 Chronicles from Mount Saint Mary's proudly noted that a number of patients had entered pottery, bead and leather work, knitting, crocheting, and hand-weaving in a hobby show at the YMCA.[65]

The inclusive, community-based ethos of recreation made it easy for administrators to call on volunteers to transform professional ideals into institutional reality. The gender profile of voluntary workers mirrored their professional colleagues. Professionals writing about voluntary workers in old age homes inevitably refer to them with the feminine pronoun. The older middle-class female tradition of friendly visiting to infirm and impoverished elderly was incorporated into the agenda of the new social work professionals. Women were expected to provide the volunteer labour needed to organize hobbies and recreational activities in homes for the elderly.[66]

Although provincial administrators were uneasy about the power base created at Marpole by the energetic Women's Auxiliary, health care journals and government reports alike stressed the need for volunteers within homes for the aged: "Friendly visitors are much needed in work with older people in nursing homes, chiefly because their lives tend to dreariness and they are confined to four walls and are often forgotten."[67] The 1949 annual report of the provincial Department of Health and Welfare noted that "[m]unicipal homes and those operated by organisations usually have very active women's auxiliaries which look after the needs of the old people."[68]

Chronic illness and recreational therapy were both the diagnosis and the prescribed cure for the elderly of the immediate post-war period. Before the development of dramatic surgical therapies for older people, interest in the aged among health professionals was mostly the remit of occupational therapists and physiotherapists. Social workers, encouraged by new sociological theories about disengagement and activism in the senescence, moved into the field of old age as well. The old age home proved to be an excellent setting for the development of these professional activities. Henceforth, the ideal care in the old age home was to be therapeutic rather than custodial.

PROFESSIONAL AGEISM AND THE IDEAL PATIENT

The professional spirit embedded in the emerging specialities of geriatric medicine and social work was a curious hybrid, a kind of Dr Jekyll and Mr Hyde figure. The women and men who were professionally involved in the process outlined in this chapter believed that they were creating a more compassionate institutional home for old people. Many were committed to a reformed institution on both a professional and personal level, seeing themselves as crusaders in the drive to divorce the old age home from its poor law past. As one UBC social work student proclaimed in a 1950 master's thesis, professionals had a responsibility to ensure that institutions for the aged were transformed into treatment centres.[69]

But there were also sharply negative facets to this new cultural focus on the aged. Placed within a box labelled "old," patients and clients were now seen and judged within the professional paradigm of "aged," reducing the potential for them to be viewed as individuals. Professional writing of the period is rife with profoundly ageist comments: elderly men and women are often presented as infirm, demanding, and resistant to change.[70] It was this attitude, as much as concerns about the vulnerability of the aged, that led credence to the notion that incarceration in an institution separated from the rest of society was appropriate for elderly men and women. Health and welfare professionals in British Columbia during the 1940s and 1950s seem to have had little interest in keeping old people in their own homes, a situation that stands in direct contrast to the United Kingdom.[71]

Institutionalization of the aged was clearly considered preferable to finding a home with kin. Health professionals and administrators believed that grandparents were an unhealthy element in the post-Second World War household, creating serious difficulties within the family because of physical and mental infirmities.[72] When UBC social work student Elizabeth Talker conducted a study of services for elderly couples in 1956, she wrote that the elderly simply did not fit into the modern family and that dependence of the aged upon their offspring would create conflict. Describing the elderly as "hyper-critical, prying, superior," Talker noted that the elderly had the lowest capacity to adapt to new life circumstances.[73] Popular culture in North America also broadcast the message that old people had no place in the extended family. American historian of old age W.A. Achenbaum notes that the elderly were simply absent from depictions of the American family in television shows, movies, and bestsellers of the day.[74]

Many social workers inside the walls of old age homes undoubtedly treated their elderly clients with compassion and kindness, but there is a striking tendency to pathologize the behaviour and conditions of the aged in the medical and social work writing of the period. For example, a 1952 report detailing the need for a medical social worker at the Marpole infirmary argued that arthritis caused emotional changes in people serious enough to warrant social work care. Arthritis, a common complaint among Marpole's elderly residents, became a psychological as well as a physical problem.[75]

Kind or cruel, these professional people nevertheless had a very clear vision of the ideal resident for the new old age home that they were fashioning. Drawn into a new paradigm where they were no longer inmates, residents of institutions for the elderly were reconceptualized as patients in need of medical and social work attention. The lives, values, and attitudes of elderly men and women were scrutinized through the professional lens of the doctor, social worker, occupational therapist, or physiotherapist. Under the earlier workhouse model, a good inmate was one who conformed to the rules and regulations of the institution. Now, an ideal patient was sociable, part of the institutional "family," and willing and able to participate in therapeutic and recreational activities (see figure 2).

The new programs, in fostering new expectations of how aged men and women would perform in residential facilities, pathologized behaviours viewed as anti-social. Professional journals urged caregivers to encourage the elderly to keep up old hobbies or develop new interests.[76] Contemporary social work thinking held that group work was both healthy and "normal." In the larger community this meant regular church attendance and a close relationship with kin.[77] Inside the old age home, a "well-adjusted" elderly man or woman, social workers argued, should show an active interest in the home by participating in social and recreational events. Current studies of old age homes have found that residents labelled "well-adjusted" by professionals are those who demonstrate the right combination of normative behaviour and

Figure 2
Institutional structures, old and new

Old Institutional Structures	
Gatekeepers	Police, Government Agents, Relief Workers
Staff	Orderlies, Administrative Superintendent, Matron or Wife
Input	Charitable groups

New Institutional Structures	
Gatekeepers	Social Workers, Physicians
Staff	Orderlies, Registered Nurses, Superintendent
Input	Occupational therapists, Physiotherapists, Nutritionists, Auxiliary

independence: knitting a tea-cosy for an exhibition and making their own way to the supper table, for example.[78]

We can see the historical roots of this professional belief system in B.C.'s old age homes of the 1940s and 1950s. Studying Taylor Manor in 1952, social work student Dennis Guest chastised residents who chose to remain in their own rooms, reading or listening to the radio.[79] The 1942 annual report of the Welfare Institutions Board stressed the importance of encouraging residents of such facilities to remain "self helpful" through recreational activities.[80] In 1948 Mary Law, superintendent of the Marpole branch of the Provincial Infirmary, stated that "[a]rousing the patients' interest in something creative brings many benefits, including a more cheerful outlook on life on the part of the patient." Professional observers believed that the chance to fashion birdhouses or change-purses helped to counter the mood of illness and physical decline that permeated institutions like the Provincial Infirmary.[81]

The focus on treating chronic illness in old age also narrowed the definition of the ideal patient. Aged men and women whose illnesses were not treatable, or whose health failed to improve following occupational therapy or physiotherapy, did not fit the new paradigm. The interest of health care professionals, particularly medical personnel, became fixed on old people who would benefit from therapeutic intervention. As for the rest, they could be maintained in a custodial institution where they would receive compassionate care. In this fashion chronic illness divided the elderly into two categories – the treatable and those who could not be healed.

This chapter has been concerned with the carving-out of new professional territories within the old age home and with the corresponding professional mapping of the bodies and psyches of the aged. Without the voices of the aged themselves, we cannot really comprehend the impact that this process had upon the way in which elderly people saw themselves and experienced their residential environment. But we can speculate.

I want to create a fictional Marpole resident of the 1940s, a kind of composite character, so we can explore the impact that these ideas may have had on patients. I call this fictional creation Fred Glen and make him a former logger whose health had been undermined by the hard physical labour of a lifetime. So let us consider his story. Faced with increasing health problems and dwindling financial resources, Glen has no choice but to enter an institution. He is given a complete physical examination by a male physician and is interviewed at length by a female social worker. He leaves the examination room feeling old and ill. The professional terminology used by the social worker, a University of British Columbia graduate, is incomprehensible to him, reminding him of welfare officers he encountered in Depression relief lines. He regards her with great suspicion.[82]

The new resident finds the whole ambience of the old age home very different from what he was used to at his cabin down by the docks. Accustomed to socializing with other single male comrades in the comfort of an alehouse, hands wrapped around a pint of beer, Fred Glen finds it difficult to make friends over a cup of tea in the communal sitting room. The "make-work" of occupational therapy and crafts is distasteful to a man used to bringing in a sensible pay packet from his labours. Anyway, "crafts" were what his mother and sisters did back home in Simcoe County. But Fred Glen cannot make the occupational therapist, or those fine auxiliary ladies, understand his point of view.

In a sense Fred Glen is an anachronism in an institution that now sees itself as middle class and therapeutic. He is not the new senior citizen meant to sit in comfortable chairs in pastel painted rooms. Never married and a transient coastal logger for much of his life, Fred is uncomfortable with the trappings of a middle-class family home. Nor is he keen to participate in the group activities of the institution. He would much prefer to listen to ball games on his transistor radio set. The only place where the new professionalism of the institution makes sense to him is at the regular physiotherapy treatments that ease his chronic back pain.

I do not want to use our Fred Glen to paint an entirely negative picture of ageist professionals invading the old age home. Ageism, like racism or sexism, is a complex phenomenon, and far too pervasive in our society to be applied so narrowly. Yet social workers, doctors, and other professionals involved in old age homes were in positions to enact broader societal prejudices against the elderly. They had the power to make important judgments concerning the lives and destinies of residents of old age homes, and were in a position to prescribe appropriate codes of personal behaviour and social interaction. This was not simply a power imbalance, but a professional mindset that sought to instill normative practice rather than accommodate individual behaviour. My research suggests that professionals were willing to make use of these powers, sometimes in ways that were not in the best interests of elderly men and women. As American medical historian Paul Starr notes, individuals in institutions are much more dependent on professionals than are people living in the community.[83] It follows that they are much more vulnerable in the face of professional power.

The 1940s and 1950s were the key period in the transformation of public facilities for aged British Columbians from custodial welfare institutions to middle-class, therapeutic nursing homes. This shift was rooted in a mélange of larger changes: public concern about poverty in old age; the growing dominance of the middle-class nuclear family; a new focus on the aged among health and social welfare professionals; and a belief in the curative potential of occupational and recreational therapy. By the close of this period, institutions for the aged were expected to be "homes" rather than simply stark facilities to house elderly indigents. This evolution opened the way for the old age home to become a socially acceptable middle-class institution.

Some elements of this change were cosmetic. Older facilities were renamed and redecorated, incorporating elements of the middle-class family home whenever institutional reality permitted. But medical science and welfare professionalism was also an integral part of the shift from poor law institution to nursing home. Standardized medical and social work procedures were implemented. Inmates were reconceptualized as patients, seen now through the therapeutic lens of social workers, nutritionists, and physiotherapists. While development varied from one institution to another, there was generally a new expectation that old age homes should provide recreational activities for residents. Volunteer and professional women played a pivotal role in providing this new kind of care to elderly patients.

The ideal patient in the reformed old age home was an elderly man or woman who was willing and able to fit the new professional agenda. This meant that he or she must have a medical or social condition that would respond to the ministrations of social work and health care staff. But equally important was the inclusion of aged residents within the "family" of the old age home: participation in appropriate social and recreational activities was another measure of good physical and mental health in old age. Sociability had become a psycho-medical category. Through prescriptive notions that set out appropriate institutional codes of behaviour and personal values, compassion was compromised by professional ageism. In terms of physical comfort, the lives of the old age home inhabitants had certainly improved immeasurably since the time of the Poor Law institutions, but it could be argued that the strict rules governing appropriate behaviour that had been so characteristic of those earlier institutions had only been substituted by more subtle discipline. There is not a huge difference, for example, between an obedient inmate and a well-behaved patient (figure 2).

The tale of Fred Glen pushes one to pose the question – how successful were professionals in implementing their new agenda for the old age home? In 1947 Mrs Wilks, an occupational therapist, attended an administrative meeting at the Home for Aged and Infirm Ladies. Noting that Wilks did not suggest any definite plans and deciding that "it did not seem the ladies in the home required such a person," the committee sent the prospective professional packing.[84] Although Marpole was much praised for its occupational therapy program, a 1953 survey decided that care given within the facility was primarily custodial in nature and therefore little professional expertise was required.[85] Similarly, a 1958 study of the Victoria Nursing Home found that the majority of residents in the institution were custodial cases because the hospital administration was unable to attract chronically ill patients.[86]

Professional ideals were also undermined within institutions by administrators and caregivers who resisted new methods of dealing with residents. At the Marpole branch of the Provincial Infirmary, B.C.'s most progressive public facility, Mary Law, superintendent from 1946, repeatedly resisted directives to create a strict staff hierarchy with specific tasks assigned to those with appropriate credentials. Law, a trained nurse, transgressed lines of authority and professional barriers by maintaining personal contact with all patients and taking on tasks assigned to the professional jurisdiction of social workers, not administrators. She earned the wrath of provincial administrators, but her patients loved her.[87] New ideas and initiatives concerning old age homes must therefore be viewed in terms of both prescription and praxis. The ideal, in terms of policy, practice, and patients, was not always attained.

Yet there were significant changes. Social workers, nutritionists, occupational therapists and physiotherapists became part of the professional community of the old age home. Residents of institutions for the elderly were now regarded as patients, both frail and deserving of care, and appropriate participants in therapeutic regimes. The old age "home" was to approximate a middle-class dwelling, with residents who were now expected to be part of an institutional "family." If the poorhouse had not entirely been discarded, at least some of its trappings had been left behind.

4 Institutional Culture: The World of the Old Age Home

Entering an old age home is a transitional moment in the life cycle, but has none of the positive possibilities of other rites of passage like marriage, giving birth, or receiving your first pay packet. What kind of institutional world awaited those who became residents of the old age home through the period of this study? And what meaning did the institutional community take within the hearts and minds of its residents? Reactions to the institutional experience were, of course, highly individualized. For some, especially single working-class men, elements of institutional life echoed previous experiences in boarding homes and logging camps. The discipline, daily routine, and ranks of other inmates may have been unwelcome, but they were likely familiar. For other old people who had left behind an independent life that included a beloved house, garden, and community, the change might have been too great ever to find a valid "home" in the institutional world.[1] But for all, the process meant they left behind one life and became part of a new community, an institutional world of old age in which power rested with administrators and caregivers, be they kind, cruel, or simply indifferent.

As we have seen, residential facilities for older British Columbians built in the late nineteenth and early twentieth centuries were based on poor law principles and practices. Deserving and impoverished inmates were given adequate accommodation, and in return they had to behave in a respectable manner and do whatever work they were capable of performing. Even charitable facilities like Victoria's Home for Aged and Infirm Ladies, and the ad hoc arrangements made for old men at the Vancouver General Hospital, were essentially run on these lines.

As I outlined in the previous chapter, during the 1940s and 1950s health and social welfare professionals in B.C. and elsewhere envisioned a new kind of old age home, a place with a warm, home-like ambience and professional medical care. In reality, these elements were not characteristic of B.C.'s residential accommodation for the elderly, even during the post-Second World War shift toward a universal welfare state. Instead, rules and routine imposed from above shaped the parameters of daily institutional life, reinforcing the historical lineage that bound public homes for aged people to poor law institutions. However, the harsh punitive regimes characteristic of central Canadian workhouses do not appear to have been the norm in B.C. In most cases, institutional ageism was more benign. There is considerable documentation of kindness and compassion by administrators and caregivers in facilities in the western province.

We should not see these elders as powerless, passive victims of fate, ill health, and poverty.[2] If they worked so hard to stay out of the institution, we can assume that they developed equally creative strategies for coping with the prescriptive culture of the old age home. Resistance took many forms, including violence, back talk, and obstinacy. Inmates also incorporated into the institutional world their life experience outside the old age home, bringing with them skills and talents, and finding companionship and pleasure as they had in their youth. In all, institutional culture was a rich medley of high drama, dull routine, punishment, and the harsh realities of poverty, illness, and death.

Old age homes in B.C. had clearly defined institutional populations. Gender, class, place of residence, state of health, and ethnicity were all factors that determined what institution an elderly person might enter. Some facilities, like the Marpole infirmary, had always catered for the bedridden and infirm. Through the 1940s, however, as old age pensions offered a greater bid for independent living, institutional populations became more infirm and frail. People no longer came into the old age home to live, but to die. Inmates became patients. They stopped taking lengthy absences from the institution and were less capable of doing work on the premises. Older patterns of seasonal use of the old age home and institutional labour died out and were replaced by medical therapies and death.

The middle-class charitable impulse that linked community and institution continued unchanged, but the evolving institutional clientele meant that, by the middle decade of the twentieth century, the old age home had become increasingly divorced from the broader community. Before old age homes became institutions for the infirm aged, residents were often recognized personalities in the local community. This, coupled with the seasonal use of some institutions, broke down the divide between the institution and the community. By 1950, however, the old age home had become a place apart, a world into which staff and visitors entered and left, but which shut residents out from former lives, locales, and connections. The case of the Home for Aged and Infirm Ladies (Rose Manor) suggests ways in which the family was incorporated into the institutional dynamic, a pattern that I see as pointing toward the future old age home.

I begin this chapter by describing institutional populations from the late nineteenth to the mid-twentieth century, noting gender, race, age, and health characteristics. I then turn to a lengthy analysis of the legacy of the Poor Law in these facilities, focusing in turn on regulation and punishment, inmate labour, and the seasonal use of institutions. This is followed by a discussion of inmate discontent and resistance and of the emotional territory of death, a near inevitability in the old age home. The final sections of the chapter set the old age home in a wider context, first by looking at the role played by the families of residents at the Home for Aged and Infirm Ladies and then by considering the changing place of the old age home in the local community.

INSTITUTIONAL POPULATIONS: GENDER, CLASS, ETHNICITY, AGE, AND HEALTH

From the perspective of gender, the demography of B.C.'s state institutions for the elderly in the first half of the twentieth century was an historical aberration. As we saw earlier, central Canadian, American, and British facilities were becoming dominated by elderly women,[3] but B.C.'s old age homes held an old poor law pattern of a majority male clientele. This was linked, of course, to the larger population characteristics and socio-economic factors described in chapter 1. Inside the Provincial Home for Old Men and Victoria's Old Men's Home was the earlier, pioneering male population of the province, now old and in need of sheltered accommodation.

In other respects institutional population patterns in B.C. conformed to changes that were taking place elsewhere. Taking the period from the late nineteenth century to the middle of the twentieth century as a whole, there are significant shifts in the composition of public and charitable facilities for the elderly: residents became older and more infirm. Younger people remained a part of some institutional communities, but they were an increasingly small group.

The public old age home in B.C. was essentially a male world. The Old Men's Home in Victoria, the Provincial Home in Kamloops, and the Allco branch of the Provincial Infirmary were occupied solely by male residents. Women rarely crossed the threshold of these facilities. At the Kamloops and Victoria institutions, managers were usually married. From the Depression until the last years of the Second World War the manager's wife and two daughters lived at the Old Men's Home in Victoria. Allco, situated in the bush outside the small Fraser Valley community of Haney, was almost entirely isolated from the world of women and families. There, the female occupational therapist who visited weekly during the 1940s was likely the only woman to enter the grounds of the facility.[4] For many residents of these institutions, the preponderance of males would simply have mirrored the gendered world of logging camps and mining communities in which they had lived their lives.

Even at institutions that catered for both sexes, there were always many more men than women. The Old People's Home in Vancouver, for example, built as a mixed sex institution, allowed space for only eleven women among a total bed capacity of sixty-eight.[5] In 1930, fifteen years after the new Home had been constructed, there were still only twelve women to the fifty male residents. Similarly, at the Marpole branch of the Provincial Infirmary 759 men were admitted between 1923 and 1939 while only 251 women became patients during the same period. In 1945, males still dominated the patient population at Marpole and were twice as numerous as women at Mount Saint Mary's, the other mixed sex infirmary institution.[6] Boarding homes for the elderly also had a considerably higher proportion of men than women. In 1948 men comprised two-thirds of the approximately 500 aged people living in Vancouver's registered boarding homes.[7]

Most of the male inmates and patients at public institutions had been blue-collar workers, a typical residential population in poor law institutions, which housed cast-offs from the capitalist labour force.[8] Provincial Home inmate registers spanning from 1900 to 1950 show that labouring and semi-skilled men made up the bulk of residents. These men came from all over the province, from Prince George, Grand Forks, Crow's Nest Pass, Salmon Arm, Parksville, Sugar Lake, Lumby, Sicamous, and Abbotsford.[9] Of the 351 applicants accepted into Victoria's Old Men's Home in the same period, almost all listed blue-collar occupations: labourers, janitors, carpenters, fishers, farmers, and sailors.[10] Urban industrial and clerical workers dominated the patient population at Marpole. Men who had worked in remote regions of the province as loggers, fishers, and miners were generally placed at Allco.[11]

The only definitely "female" old age home in the province was the Home for Aged and Infirm Ladies. The venerable institution took only women patients, was administered by a committee of women, and was

staffed by women. The sole exceptions to this gender dominance were
a string of Chinese kitchen help, the gardener, and the men who stoked
the furnace. Early patient registers from the Home for Aged and Infirm
Ladies and the minute books of the Home Committee show that,
although most residents were from the local area, applications came
from as far away as Edmonton and California. Names of residents
noted in the minute books indicate that the populace was fairly
homogenous: white and Christian. A Jewish woman entering in 1907
was specifically commented upon in the committee minutes, as was a
black woman two years later.[12]

Old age was moving toward being seen as an entirely separate stage
of the life cycle, but we see vestiges of traditional poor law patterns
in the inclusion of younger people within some institutional populations.[13] Before provincial bureaucrats sharpened their regulatory gaze
on facilities for the aged in the late 1930s, single mothers and babies
sometimes resided in smaller charitable homes and private hospitals.
These institutions typically had a range of clients, young and old. In
1933 the proprietor of Victoria's Maple Rest Nursing Home stated
emphatically that she "did not take babies as they could not be mixed
with old people." Nonetheless, occasional babies and young children
were cared for at her establishment.[14]

Middle-aged disabled and chronically ill men and women were a
significant proportion of the patient community at Marpole. Among
a total patient population of 175, Isobel Harvey found 111 people
under sixty years living at this branch of the Provincial Infirmary in
1945, a reflection of the dual use of that institution as an old age home
and a residence for the physically disabled.[15] Patient statistics from
Victoria's Chinese Hospital reflect a similar dichotomy. In 1942 the
residents at the Chinese Hospital were divided equally into two groups,
with five in the forty to sixty-nine-year-old category and seven listed
as seventy years or older.[16] Although the elderly comprised the majority of the patient population at the facilities used by the City of
Vancouver to house public patients, 19 per cent of residents at the
Glen Hospital, Grandview Hospital, and Heather Street Annex Hospital were under sixty in 1948. At Allco, however, the population was
clearly aged: in 1949 the average age of the residents was seventy-six
years. Similarly, of the 132 men admitted to Victoria's Old Men's
Home between 1935 and 1950, only three were under sixty years of
age. The Home for Aged and Infirm Ladies clearly catered for elderly
women: there were 108 residents over seventy in December 1942, and
only four women in the forty to sixty-nine age group.[17]

At any given time, public old age homes in the province reflected the
general ethnic composition of B.C.'s population. Before the First World

War the character of the Old Men's Home in Victoria was decidedly British: in both 1908 and 1913 more than half of the residents were from the United Kingdom.[18] The majority of the early residents at the Home for Aged and Infirm Ladies were also from England, Scotland, Wales, and Ireland, as were their male counterparts in the Provincial Home. Certainly, British working-class inmates would have equated public old age homes with the detested poorhouse they had known in their homeland: references to "the poorhouse" are common in correspondence relating to men from the United Kingdom.[19]

By the end of the Second World War, however, the ethnicity of the Kamloops institution had definitely broadened, and patient rolls from the Provincial Infirmary (Marpole branch) in 1948 included people born in Germany, Sweden, China, Switzerland, and Italy. First Nations people appear to have been a very small percentage of the total number of patients: between 1942 and 1955 only three aboriginal people were admitted to Marpole. Full maintenance costs for this group of patients, minus old age pension payments, were paid by the federal government's Department of Indian Affairs.[20]

As detailed in chapter 2, a small number of ethnic homes for the aged provided accommodation for specific ethnic groups. The oldest of these was the Chinese Hospital in Victoria, established in 1884. This facility took only men, reflecting the gender imbalance in the local Chinese community. A second home for elderly Chinese men operated in New Westminster in the 1920s.[21] Scandanavian groups were quick to take advantage of government funding for old age homes in the late 1940s. A decade later, elderly Danes, Swedes, and Icelanders could enter facilities established by their own ethnic groups in Vancouver.[22]

Overall, the character of residential populations in B.C.'s old age homes remained relatively stable in terms of gender, age, and ethnicity over the period under study. What did change, however, was the health of people living in these institutions. Public homes for the province's aged were not originally intended to provide nursing care for the infirm elderly. The evidence of the 1903 commission of investigation into the Provincial Home for Old Men makes it clear that inmates were expected to be fit and capable of working for their keep.[23] In the first decades of operation, administrators at the Old Men's Home turned away sick applicants. In 1917 the Home Committee explicitly stated that "the Home is not a Home for Incurables, even if they are aged, and infirm."[24] This situation had altered considerably by the Second World War. In 1943 George Havard, manager of the Old Men's Home, noted that inmates were increasingly physically incapacitated: "Prior to the Old Age Pension scheme, out-side relief, etc., there were always a few inmates active and willing to perform routine tasks in the Home. The inmates of today are definitely totally incapacitated, therefore unable to help, leaving the upkeep of the Home to the staff."[25]

As the war continued, administrators at the Provincial Infirmary also noted a pattern of increasing numbers of bed patients.[26] The 1943, 1948, and 1950 annual reports all commented on the great demand for bed care at Marpole, a situation that had apparently existed for some time. In 1956 Marpole's superintendent reiterated the now familiar refrain in her annual report: "I would like to emphasise the fact again that the patients we are admitting to Mount St. Mary's and Allco are much more helpless than in previous years, requiring a great deal more time and care."[27] Isobel Harvey's 1945 survey of public old age homes in B.C. found that the twenty-bed hospital unit at Allco, meant to care for temporary cases, was being used for permanent patients because there was no room for them at other branches of the Provincial Infirmary. Harvey also noted that the Provincial Home had become an infirmary for aged men.[28]

As discussed in the first chapter, this shift was rooted in the 1927 Old Age Pensions Act, which granted a small monthly pension to British subjects over seventy years of age with limited means. Throughout the 1930s and 1940s the numbers of elderly British Columbians being granted pensions or other forms of social assistance increased substantially.[29] Many elderly men and women who would have been forced to enter an old age home were able to delay or avoid entering an institution. The implementation of the 1937 provincial Hospital Clearances program, designed to remove the chronically ill from acute care hospital beds and described more fully in the next chapter, also served to increase the population of the frail elderly in old age homes. In Victoria, as part of the new scheme, eight men were transferred from the Jubilee Hospital Annex to the Old Men's Home in the spring of 1938. It is certain that these men were in poorer health than the general population of the Home at this time. Superintendent Havard described the eight as "total disability cases" and "nursing cases" in subsequent reports, and the Home Committee hired an orderly to care for them. The presence of an orderly, the first staff member at the institution hired specifically to care for infirm inmates, may also have changed the character of the inmate population. A year later Havard noted that it was no longer necessary to transfer ailing inmates to nursing homes, signalling a fundamental shift in policy regarding the Home's clientele.[30]

Residential populations of old age homes are instrumental in determining institutional culture and character. The class and gender profile of B.C.'s old age homes, with large numbers of single, working-class men, reinforced ties with older poor law institutional facilities. The continued presence of a significant number of British residents also bound B.C.'s homes for elderly people to the poorhouse, a link that was undoubtedly enhanced by the particular hatred with which the English working classes regarded that institution. Middle-class family values and medical and social welfare professionalism were not part of the world in which they had lived their working lives. The mixed ages of residents at other institutions also harkened back to earlier forms of accommodation where older residents were not set apart but incorporated into a diverse institutional community. In ethnic old age homes and Victoria's Home for Aged and Infirm Ladies the institutional community was more homogeneous and the charitable impulse stronger. In these facilities patients were united by race in the first instance and by gender and respectability in the second.

Over the inter-war years the population of old age homes began to change from a relatively healthy group to an infirm clientele. As the numbers of frail and bed ridden patients grew, institutional routine and culture and patterns of institutionalization also changed. As American historian Carole Haber has noted, during the first half of the twentieth century a hospital atmosphere came to prevail in residential homes for the aged.[31] Inmates became patients, increasingly in need of medical care. An institutional economy that was dependent on patient labour evolved into one that relied on pension income. The use of the old age home on a seasonal or occasional basis declined and patient culture became more focused around the limits of infirm old age and the inevitability of death. Single labouring men, less able to reconnect with their old communities or to practice working-class skills and customs inside the old age home, became classless "patients." Punitive regimes, never a prominent aspect of the old age home in B.C., became less appropriate. By the 1940s administrators were noticeably kind to their ailing charges.

POOR LAW PRINCIPLES: REGULATIONS AND PUNISHMENT

The heritage of the workhouse was strongest in public homes for the aged, where regulations were steeped in the ethos of the Poor Law. The process of applying to enter one of these facilities, with lengthy forms to be completed, and a formal interview in the case of Victoria, established the hierarchical power relationship into which inmates were entering. Henceforth, civic and institutional administrators and, later, health and social welfare professionals would determine the fortunes of the aged applicant. Detailed information concerning family, state of health, assets, and former and current places of residence was

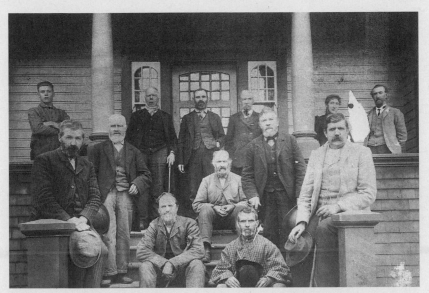

Residents and staff at the Provincial Home for Aged Men, Kamloops, 1898. A rare image of inmates and staff at the provincial institution that housed some of the "surplus men" of the province. Inmates of this period were expected to be fit and capable of working for their keep, and some left the Home to live independently during the mild months of the year and returned with the cold weather. (British Columbia Provincial Archives)

required. Once the applicant's life had been set out on the printed form, and perhaps also in medical and social reports, character was scrutinized and need assessed by state authorities. In exchange for shelter, food, and care in their aging years, applicants gave up the basic tenants of citizenship – the right to personal privacy and the right to determine where and how they would live.

The Poor Law principle of less eligibility set the basis for entry into these facilities. At the Old People's Home in Vancouver, and the Old Men's Home in Victoria and its brother institution in Kamloops, inmates were meant to be destitute. Anything the applicants owned of value was turned over to the state.[32] John Elbridge, a seventy-five-year-old labourer who entered Victoria's civic facility in 1920, relinquished his house and lot.[33] Public patients at the Royal Oak Private Hospital gave the municipality pension money or income from rental property.[34] At the Provincial Infirmaries a deceased patient's estate was charged a daily maintenance fee for the time she or he had been a patient in the institution.[35] In all cases it appears that if an inmate or patient chose to leave the institution then they would receive back money or assets, minus the cost of their upkeep.

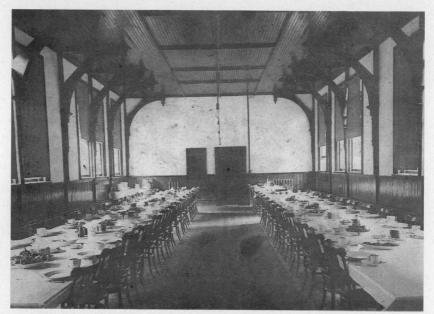

Dining room, the Provincial Home for Aged Men, Kamloops, ca 1890s. Evidence from the 1890s shows that the facility's dining room was a site of resistance and punishment. At that time the dining room was the main communal area in the building and thus its stark and cheerless decor underscores the poor law ethos that lay behind these early public institutions for the aged. (British Columbia Provincial Archives)

Similar procedures were also the practice at private and charitable institutions, where assets could be parleyed into guarantees of care. The Home for Aged and Infirm Ladies entered into various financial agreements with prospective residents and also accepted civic cases. Private agreements usually took the shape of a lump sum or assets given over in exchange for life care. In May 1907, for instance, the Home Committee accepted $500 from a Victoria spinster entering the Home. The remainder of the woman's estate was to be received when she died.[36] This arrangement appears to have been concluded on a mutually acceptable basis before the woman came into the Home. But other agreements, arrived at after a woman had been resident for a time, have overtones of strong coercion. In 1915, for instance, the committee agreed to allow a resident to remain for $12 per month if a legal document was drawn up entitling the institution to the balance of money owed when the woman's house was sold.[37]

Impersonal institutional regimentation took away the right to order one's life as one chose. Routine schedules allowed for a high level of administrative surveillance and facilitated the tasks of institutional housekeeping and patient care.[38] Daily life in Victoria's Old Men's Home, for example, was regulated with a 7:30 am dressing bell, breakfast at eight am, dinner at noon, supper at five pm, and lights out at nine pm, when, as the superintendent reported in 1893, "all the lights must be out and silence reign supreme."[39] This description dates from the turn of the century, but the imposition of a rigid timetable was a feature of life in public facilities throughout the first half of the twentieth century as well, another similarity with the workhouse and other social control institutions. Such practices were also the norm at old age homes that had no direct institutional lineage to the poorhouse. At the Home for Aged and Infirm Ladies, a 1907 committee ruling stated that breakfast be served at 9 am, dinner at 1 pm, and that all able residents must come to the table for each meal. In 1916 lights out time was extended from 9 to 10 pm.[40] Boarding homes of the 1940s, which housed elderly men and women most capable of independent living, also set rules regulating lights out and bathing times. Residents were permitted one bath each week at a set time, a limitation that would have been a particular hardship for those who suffered from incontinence.[41]

Other administrative practices also robbed inmates of personal dignity and choice. Residents at the Old Men's Home in Victoria were provided with new clothing in the 1920s and public charges were not required to wear the shapeless garments that set English inmates apart when they ventured outside the poorhouse,[42] but a grim custom of using cast-off clothing from undertakers for inmates was followed at several institutions caring for public patients. Mrs Ross, proprietor of the Maple Rest Nursing Home in the 1930s, dressed former hospital patients with clothing donated by Hayward's Funeral Parlour.[43] Elderly residents at Mount Saint Mary's in the 1950s were dressed in clothing left with bodies at the funeral parlour but not required by the undertaker.[44] Imagine the emotional impact this symbolic act must have had on the elderly inmates, laying aside their own worn clothes in exchange for garments meant for the grave.

Another aspect of the Poor Law ethic, which was apparent in both public and private homes for the aged, was an emphasis on moral behaviour and respectability. Applicants to the Old Men's Home had to submit two references from "reputable residents" of Victoria. Regulation 6 of the Provincial Home, a document signed by inmates when they entered the facility, stated that "[t]he inmates of the Home are required to be clean in their persons and habits and to do their utmost to keep up the respectability and tone of the establishment."[45] Character and respectability were also important at the Home for Aged and Infirm Women, where a delegation from the Home Committee interviewed prospective applicants. In 1904 one applicant was accepted on the condition that she be "made cleaner by some friends interested in her."[46] A resident was asked to leave in 1910 because of bad language and inappropriate conduct.[47] Staff at the women's facility were also expected to be of good moral character. In 1909, after some discussion about the conduct of one female staff member, it was decided that male callers could only be entertained one night per week and that this should take place in the office rather than the small parlour.[48] In 1941 instructions were posted in the Nurses' Home stating that gentlemen visitors were not allowed on the premises except in the sitting room.[49]

Elderly residents at these facilities were meant to be morally upstanding citizens and to follow the rules of the institution, an attempt to ensure that public charity was given to only the deserving aged poor. Middle-class codes of inmate and patient behaviour usually remained unaltered from the historical moment at which the institution was founded.[50] At the Old Men's Home and the Provincial Home the rules stated that inmates were not permitted to leave the premises without permission from the manager, use profane language, or bring alcohol into the institution. At both facilities the superintendent had the right to prohibit "undesirable" friends from visiting.[51]

We cannot know how closely written rules were followed at these two institutions. Efforts to mould inmates into responsible institutional citizens were mediated by the fact that administrators were dealing with elderly men, some in poor health or with disabilities, who had nowhere else to go. Many of the men who were expelled simply ended up back in the facility several weeks or months later. Moreover, the fit between "respectable" middle-class morality and "rough" male working-class culture was often poor: a significant number of inmates had little regard for social niceties like polite language. The manager of the Old Men's Home in Victoria in the early twentieth century was more concerned with whether it would be necessary to call out the police patrol wagon than with the manners of his inmates.[52]

Punishment at B.C.'s two public homes for old men was not nearly so harsh as it was at houses of industry and houses of refuge elsewhere in Canada. There, incarceration in punishment cells, fines, and permanent expulsions were still used to subdue unruly inmates in the 1930s and 1940s.[53] Nonetheless, the principles of discipline and respect for authority seem to have been important ones. Superintendents routinely expelled inmates for refusing to obey orders, for bad language, and for behaviour they deemed unsuitable.[54] At Kamloops, when Superintendent McLean was in charge during the early years of the twentieth century, erring inmates had their meal plates taken away. The loss of the plate meant that the resident had forfeited the right to be part of

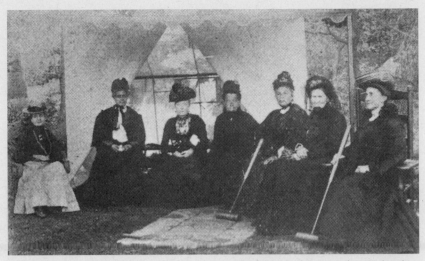

Miss Roblee, matron (on left), with early group of inmates at the Home for Aged and Infirm Ladies, no date. Another image from an early history of the Victoria institution, showing staff and residents of the Home. The genteel image of these ladies, some holding croquet mallets, all respectably dressed, demonstrates the elevated character of the women's institution. (British Columbia Provincial Archives)

the institutional community until the issue between inmate and superintendent was satisfactorily resolved.[55] The use of food as a punishment or a reward was common in English workhouses as well, where, like at B.C.'s public homes for the aged, the consumption of food assumed overarching importance in the narrow confines of the institutional community.[56]

Authority at the Home for Aged and Infirm Ladies rested in the first instance with the matron. The management committee of the Home invariably supported the matron in confrontations with residents. In October 1914 Miss Brett was told that "she must positively refrain from interfering with the matron's perogative or will be summarily ejected from the home."[57] Two years later, when the matron reported that Mrs Frank of Rossland was being "most insolent in the dining room to her," the committee decided to interview Mrs Frank and stress the importance of being respectful to the staff and the matron.[58] The establishment certainly found it necessary and desirable to have a clear code of behaviour and make it known to the residents. In 1918 copies of the newly revised rules were printed and posted in each room.[59]

Poor Law principles were deeply etched into the culture of B.C.'s public old age homes and were also evident in charitable and private facilities. A range of administrative practices underscored this philosophy. New residents had to prove both need and eligibility for assistance.

They were forced to reveal intimate details of their bodies and their life histories. Institutional regulations limited personal choice and set a daily timetable governing residents' lives. These practices, characteristics of Goffman's "total" institutional paradigm, stripped those entering the old age home of power and status, establishing the authority of health and social work professionals and institutional administrators to judge, to give, and to take away.[60]

POOR LAW PRACTICES: INMATE LABOUR

Another facet of life at B.C.'s public homes for the aged that reflected poorhouse philosophy, particularly in the years before residents became more frail, was the role played by patient labour in the institutional economy. But here again, institutional regimes were clearly more benign than for those residing in workhouses in central Canada or for younger men at Depression relief camps. Elderly men and women in B.C.'s public old age homes were not required to undertake useless work or to labour without tools.[61] Under the direction of the superintendent, they did all kinds of work to help with institutional housekeeping and improvement. This labour, compulsory for all healthy inmates, was another way in which administrative power and surveillance were reinforced within the institutional community.

Residents at the Old People's Home in Vancouver were expected to perform some kind of work as long as they were able to do so. Early reports show that inmate labour produced enough vegetables to feed the residents for much of the year, a fact that lends credence to the report that the institution operated a farm in the early years. Inmates did gardening, housework, and general labour. Residents at the two public homes for old men did "male" work, using skills gained during their labouring years. At Victoria's civic home inmates who were physically capable worked two hours each day. They undertook minor construction projects, improved the grounds where the Home was · located, and kept the kitchen garden.[62] Provincial Home residents worked on the institution's farm, but they were also required to undertake the more "female" tasks of clearing tables, helping in the kitchen, and keeping their rooms in order.[63] Before more staff were engaged to assist with the growing numbers of frail residents, men at the public old age homes in Kamloops and Victoria undertook another "female" task, nursing fellow inmates when they fell sick. Writing to the nephew of a deceased inmate in 1923, the superintendent at the Provincial Home explained that the best of the dead man's clothes had been divided among the inmates who had written letters and cared for the man before he was transferred to the sick ward.[64]

Some inmates had jobs for which they took personal responsibility, moving into a grey area between staff and residents. During the 1920s the cook at the Old Men's Home in Victoria was also an inmate. Although he was only fifty-three years old, this man transferred his savings to the Home and took on the role of cook in exchange for a promise of care in old age.[65] At Kamloops, one black inmate told the 1903 commission, "I am head gardener, I loaded wagons of apples and they came down to the apple house, they were put in the apple house."[66] Another Kamloops inmate did the bookkeeping from the late 1920s until his death in 1936.[67]

Reliable and obliging inmates greatly assisted administrators. Miss Elwell was so helpful with nursing duties during both the day and the night at the Home for Aged and Infirm Ladies in 1913 that the management decided not to charge her one month's board.[68] David Havard, the superintendent's son at the Old Men's Home in the inter-war years, described one particularly helpful inmate: "Paddy was very much a 'willing horse' and had been a boon to my parents all those years. Kindness itself, he lavished special attention to the disadvantaged feeble old men who needed help with dressing, climbing stairs and all other difficulties confronted."[69] Moreover, the fiscal advantages of having work done by residents were significant within the institutional economy. The cherished bookkeeper at the Provincial Home was paid $27.50 per month for his work; after he died the non-inmate who replaced him requested $75 for the same task.[70]

Even when the general health of inmates in public institutions deteriorated, there continued to be an expectation that patients would perform some work for their keep. During the Depression years and into the Second World War, the Old Men's Home in Victoria was still very much dependent on inmate work, with only the manager, his wife, one cook, and an orderly to care for forty men. New institutional bylaws stated that inmates in the Home were responsible for performing work about the premises as directed by the superintendent. This was also the case at Vancouver's Old People's Home, where residents were expected to make their own beds and perform light housekeeping tasks.[71]

Although inmate labour was clearly part of the institutional power relationship it should not be viewed in an entirely negative light. As former labourers and homemakers, after all, most inmates would have had a strong self-identity as capable working people. Institutional labour might allow them to hold onto an identity forged during their working years. Hence, when the women at the Home for Aged and Infirm Ladies helped out with summer canning in the kitchen, described by Matron Alice Robb as a "family affair," they were practising valued womanly skills and doing something they knew was useful.[72]

Tools, if they had not been sold for food and shelter before admittance, might well serve a practical purpose within the old age home, shoring up a sense of self undermined by institutionalization. A set of plumbers' wrenches or a skill-saw would have been a tangible link to a man's personal heritage as a working man in the larger community. At the Old Men's Home in Victoria a former scissors and knife sharpener made good use of his sharpening barrow in his new home. Inmates also recreated the ambience of their trade within the world of the institution. A former fruit peddler bought bunches of bananas and distributed them in the Home, to the delight of the young children who lived there.[73]

Opportunities to work outside the old age home also allowed elderly inmates at the Provincial Home and the Old Men's Home temporary escape from the physical confines of institution. After all, many residents at these facilities, like inmates at Allco and Marpole, were accustomed to working outdoors. As one Kamloops resident stated in 1903, "I am generally outside ... I am out of doors most of the day I feel better when working."[74] In other cases, when elderly residents did extra chores for small sums of money, inmate labour found more temporal remuneration. The superintendent of the Provincial Home in the 1920s found that the chance to earn a "little pocket money" made the old men in his charge more content.[75] Residents at the Vancouver Old People's Home could also undertake additional work if they wished to earn money. Institutional budgets from the 1920s and 1930s always contained an item for "Wages, Inmates." In 1920 this amounted to nearly $1,000. The figures show a steady decline in the amount allocated to this category and a significant dip from $613 to $269 in the years between 1931 and 1939.[76]

But not all residents were happy about working, likely equating inmate labour with the hated poorhouse. Inmates interviewed for the 1903 commission believed that they were overworked, and some fiercely resented the authoritarian attitude of the superintendent.[77] In 1950 Allco residents refused to do anything to improve their bleak institutional home.[78] Other men and women must have resented being paid a token sum or nothing at all for work that they had previously have done for a good wage or in their own kitchens and homes. Institutional labour, although not set in the punitive context as it was in workhouses elsewhere, was still under the direction of the superintendent and likely continued to be regarded by some as a punishment even when it was not presented as such.[79] Men also might have felt that having to perform "female" tasks was an affront to a male identity already weakened by dependency and loss of autonomy. Unlike prisons or asylums, where a willing worker could secure early release, there was little real reward for work in old age homes.

Private and charitable facilities for the aged also expected their elderly residents to work. Patients at the Maple Rest Nursing Home in Victoria were meant to make their own beds and keep their rooms tidy. All those who lived at the Home for the Friendless in Summerland, regardless of their age, did some work in the home.[80] Elderly women residents at the Soroptimist House in Vancouver "lent a helping hand with light duties in their rooms."[81] Across the Strait of Georgia, at the Home for Aged and Infirm Ladies, residents who assisted with the work of the Home were accorded the privilege of using the kitchen when they wished. In 1910, as part of an economising effort, it was decided that all able-bodied residents who paid fifteen dollars or less per month should wait on themselves at the meal table and fetch their own hot water bottles. Women who could not cover the cost of their board at the Home sometimes did extra work in lieu of making monetary payments.[82]

Work defined the daily routine of the old age home and served to incorporate elderly inmates into the power structure of the institutional world. Some residents felt the regimentary and authoritarian character of work keenly, perhaps refusing to participate. But work also served as a way for inmates to "re-member" themselves as they were before they entered the institution. Work could be a chance to use their hands and their bodies, to be knowledgeable, to pick up their own tools and go outside the walls of the old age home. These were working people, and it makes good sense that many might use their labour to render the institutional world into a "home." Moreover, raking out potatoes at the Provincial Home's farm or canning at the Home for Aged and Infirm Ladies was real work as opposed to the make-work of occupational therapy and crafts that men find so distasteful in contemporary nursing homes. In sum, institutional labour was about the same things that non-institutional work is about – power, survival, and identity.

POOR LAW PATTERNS: ENTERING
AND LEAVING THE INSTITUTION

Another Poor Law pattern that persisted at the Provincial Home and Home for Aged and Infirm Ladies until after the Second World War was a daily or seasonal use of the institution by some residents.[83] This was one way in which inmates set their own agenda in the institutional context. Following a seasonal pattern was familiar to most from work in the resource-based industries of the province, and allowed men to hold onto partial independence in old age. A small number of women at the Victoria institution shaped their institutional lives around a similar Poor Law pattern in one of two ways: they either found some employment locally, or took holidays away from the institution to visit friends or relations. Both options allowed the women to balance independence and security. Other than relieving administrators of a small amount of maintenance costs, it is difficult to see this as a system that worked strongly in the interests of an institution.

A number of inmates at the Provincial Home used the provincial facility as a winter base, departing during the summer months or at harvest time.[84] Signing out from the institution with a couple of fellow residents, men were able to live a vagabond existence, finding piecework in seasonal industries or simply travelling around. They could visit old friends or relatives, secure in the knowledge that they had a place to return to when the weather turned cool. Jack Bell, pulled out of the waters off West Vancouver in August 1923 after he fell off the ferry, was taking his annual leave of absence.[85] In 1924 Sam Penner told the provincial police constable in Vernon that he planned to spend July and August picking berries in Naramata.[86] Four years later another inmate wrote to inform the superintendent that he would not be back before September 10th as he was needed to help with the threshing. "I am well," he concluded, "and feeling like a fighting cock."[87]

The case of James Peckham shows how one man used the Provincial Home as a winter residence over a number of years. Peckham entered the institution in August 1923. The next summer he was officially absent from July 3rd to August 30th, having returned to his last residence in the Okanagan region. In 1925 he followed the same pattern, leaving in mid-July and returning two months later. He apparently spent the summers with a friend, but probably saw his two sons, both Okanagan residents, as well. He did not take a leave of absence in the summer of 1926, likely due to worsening health, and died in early October.[88]

Seasonal use of public old age homes was an enduring custom: even as late as 1956 the waiting list for B.C.'s public institutions varied according to season. In the summer approximately twenty people were on waiting lists, while in the winter the list generally increased to one hundred men and women.[89] But seasonal use of institutions relied on the certainty that one could re-enter the old age home when the cold weather arrived, and by this point institutional accommodation was increasingly scarce. The changing character of the institutional population from inmate to patient would also have discouraged seasonal sojourns. Old men who were in reasonable health and had an old age pension cheque in their pocket could ride out the winter months as a paying guest at a Vancouver boarding house, while those inside the old age home were now too frail to consider summer sojourns.

It is clear that this seasonal use of the old age home was a male pattern. As James Snell notes, women could not hope to find the same kinds of seasonal employment. Nor were they socialized to accept the kind of rough living that men on leave from the home likely took for granted.[90] But women at the Home for Aged and Infirm Ladies also strategized to combine the security of the old age home with continued independence. Some residents took regular or periodic holidays. In March 1903, for example, Mrs Laird received permission to leave the institution for one week. In 1913 Miss Vetch took ten days' summer holiday. Mrs Harrison left in December 1918 to spend the winter in California. She was delighted with the Home, she told the committee, and hoped to return in the spring.[91]

More interesting and unexpected is the small number of women who lived at the Home for Aged and Infirm Ladies and found small amounts of regular employment in the local community. As stated at the turn of the century, administrators of the home were in agreement with this practice so long as the women in question continued to help in the home each day before going out to work. Two residents, Mrs Laird and Mrs Drew, were to be notified of this decision. Six years later Mrs Drew was still working one half day per week outside the Home. In 1910 Mrs Newton asked if she could go out to work for two weeks to earn some money for new clothing. Permission was granted.[92]

This mode of institutional living shows one way in which aged British Columbians were able to make use of the old age home to suit their needs. It also suggests that there were two groups within the institutional population: those who had the physical ability or networks of support to allow them to leave and return, and those who did not. Men such as Sam Penner at the Provincial Home and women like Mrs Harrison at the Home for Aged and Infirm Ladies would have had a very different attitude toward their institutional home than those who lived there permanently. No institution can be "total" if an inmate can come and go at her or his bequest. Mrs Laird, who left the Home for Aged and Infirm Ladies several times a week to work, likely felt a positive sense of independence each time she closed the Rupert Street door behind her. Sojourns and time away, perhaps to former habitats and communities, allowed these people to view their institutional home as a convenience rather than a prison.[93]

THE INSTITUTIONAL WORLD: DISCONTENTMENT AND RESISTANCE

To comprehend the nature of the power of patients and inmates within an institutional community we have to set aside our own notions of agency and personal satisfaction. In the more confined world of the institutionalized and the infirm aged small tasks and issues often loom larger. A similar inverse quality can be seen when we consider power

and resistance among those on the margins. For the powerless, sub-
verting authority may be a seemingly small act of dissent or even a
passive withdrawal from the institutional community: revolutionary
moments we see as insignificant can in fact be of huge importance in
the institutional context. A grumble to a visitor, leaving one's plate on
the dinner table, or wearing the same pair of socks two days in a row –
all these can constitute defiance and rejection of authority.

There were many unhappy and discontented residents in old age
homes and they were not always silent about their grievances. Some
concerns centred on the sensory assault of institutional life. Inmates
were critical of the lack of privacy and noise levels in busy and sometimes crowded institutions. Family members were asked to remove a
resident at the Home for Aged and Infirm Ladies in 1952 because of
the disturbance she was creating at nights.[94] One female patient at
Marpole wrote a bitter letter of complaint two years later, stating that
"I don't like any institution I cant stand the noise it is taking my
nerfe to pieces ..."[95] This was no idle complaint: in 1952 a handful
of Marpole patients were so noisy at night, and space so restricted,
that they had to be moved to the main hallway to allow the other
patients to sleep.[96] Staff at Marpole believed that patients also found
the enthusiastic meetings and annual rummage sales of the Women's
Auxiliary upsetting.[97]

Noise and overcrowding were not the only issues for people in old
age homes. Elderly residents also complained about the boredom of
institutional life, poor treatment, and unbearable smells.[98] Boredom
was particularly apparent in institutions where the elderly were not
healthy enough to work or able to get out into the local community.
Latter-day images of homes for the aged, where frail residents sit idle
for much of the day, convey an almost unbearable sense of lethargy
and emptiness, characteristics typical of those who live in old age
homes.[99] Allco residents must have felt especially cut off from the
outside world. Visiting the former work camp in 1950, the provincial
minister of Health and Welfare commented that, while the residents
seemed fairly content, "I was impressed by the fact that most of the
patients show no interest in their surroundings."[100] Withdrawal from
the communal world of the old age home was a clear rejection of the
agenda put forward by social workers and occupational therapists
keen to engage the elderly in crafts and group activities.

Policy adviser Isobel Harvey visited the Provincial Home in 1945
and discovered that any magazines brought into the institution simply
vanished, swept away by inmates desperate for imaginative stimulation
and news from the wider world. At Mount Saint Mary's, Harvey found
that "all [the patients] I saw were just sitting in groups talking or lying
in bed quiet." Residents suffered from loneliness, missing family and

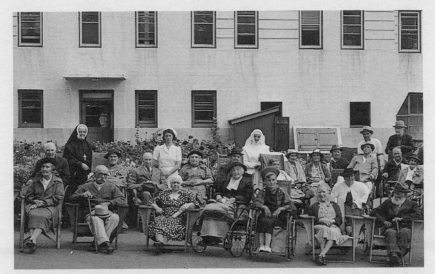

Mount Saint Mary's: hospital staff and patients, 1943. This later photograph of the residents at the Victoria branch of the Provincial Infirmary shows a much more infirm clientele gathered outside a hospital style institution designed to provide medical care for elderly men and women. The Sisters of Saint Ann were deemed appropriate caregivers for this vulnerable client group. (British Columbia Provincial Archives)

friends. Harvey, her social worker's ear in action, heard concerns about "children who fail to write or visit."[101]

In an earlier era, fit inmates did more than merely voice complaints. Daily routine was sometimes shattered by violence in the male institutions. Institutional regulations forbidding such behaviour were ignored, and frustration and anger flared. Rows erupted between inmates over card games, at the meal table, and in shared bathrooms. Reporting on a dispute with a fellow resident in 1903, one Kamloops inmate stated, "I had a fight with him in the wash room, he knocked me out with the piss pot, but I got even. Only one fight with him. I blackened his eyes."[102] Inmates, returning drunk to the Home, were insolent to their superintendent, and turned physical when restrained. It is impossible to know to whom or what this antagonistic behaviour was really directed, but these are clearly the actions of unhappy people. In 1919, one woman at the Home for Aged and Infirm Ladies committed suicide by drowning herself. Resident in the institution for only seventeen days, one can only guess at her desperate frame of mind.[103]

But such drama was a comparative rarity in old age homes. Inmate dissatisfaction was most frequently expressed in smaller acts of insubordination. The pages of the daily book kept by the superintendent at the Vancouver Old People's Home in January 1917 gives ready illustrations of how male inmates rebelled against the imposition of institutional routine and regulations. On January 5 one inmate was absent overnight without leave and another was found spitting in the ward. Two weeks later the superintendent noted that a third inmate had been out all night without permission, a fourth had declined to empty the ash and litter bins, and a fifth had been "grossly impertinent to the matron." The final inmate was clearly having a difficult time: the following day he refused to do table duty and was "insolent" to the superintendent.[104]

When Bernice Leydier was doing research on Vancouver boarding homes for the elderly in the late 1940s she found that food was both a social event and a source of real pleasure for the institutionalized aged.[105] Food was also a common point of patient resistance and dissatisfaction. Inmates complained a lot about what they had to eat. Residents at the Home for Aged and Infirm Ladies agitated about the unchanging meals in 1909, although this topic does not reappear in the committee minute books until 1948.[106] Visiting the Provincial Home in the 1940s, Isobel Harvey was struck by the way in which food had become a focus of men's lives: she reported that the inmates began lining up more than a quarter of an hour before meals were served.[107]

At the Home for Aged and Infirm Ladies resistance developed around the question of women coming to the table for meals. In 1910 Mrs Finch refused to come to her dinner, only changing her mind after two interviews with a member of the Home Committee. Two years later, with more minor instances having taken place, the Home Committee decided to charge residents who remained in their rooms for meals. In spite of this ruling this continued to be a point of tension. In 1913 three women refused to come down for meals, one going instead to the kitchen and making her own meals when she wished. A decade on the issue still simmered and management put up a notice stating that no food was allowed in bedrooms without the consent of the matron.[108]

Transcripts of the 1903 commission into the Provincial Home, formed to investigate allegations of cruelty and abuse within the institution, give us the voice of the inmates and their thoughts about authority and punishment. One man agreed that Superintendent McLean deserved some of the criticism being directed toward him, saying, "I object to his manner." However, admitted the witness, his confrontations with the superintendent were the fault of both parties. The inmate recounted that there was "a little row between us and he put me out. I had a growl with him, some dissatisfaction. If you object to work he puts you out. I do all I can some I can't do."[109] Even in the 1940s, when the professional discourse about the old age home would suggest a more liberal, compassionate attitude toward inmates and patients, residents at public institutions complained about poor treatment at the hands of staff and administrators.[110]

Alcohol use was an ongoing issue at homes for the aged and another site of patient resistance against institutional power. Inmates were not supposed to consume alcohol, but this was clearly not a realistic expectation. Reports from the Old Men's Home, the Provincial Home, and the Vancouver Old People's Home repeatedly note men returning to the homes drunk.[111] But administrators were usually lenient toward inmates who drank *outside* the premises of the old age home, perhaps recognizing that the large role of alcohol in male culture made such policing impossible. It was the consumption of alcohol *inside* the confines of the institution that most troubled administrators. As late as 1955, an investigation was undertaken at Marpole and Allco to see if there was any truth to the rumour that patients were being supplied with liquor.[112]

There was a rather different pattern for dealing with alcohol at the Home for Aged and Infirm Ladies. Going outside the institution to drink, which would compromise both female and institutional respectability, was strictly forbidden. However, women were allowed to consume alcohol in their rooms on some occasions. The minutes make it clear that some women had problems meeting these limitations. In 1903 it was decided that Mrs Gladwell be permitted one small drink in the evening. One year later, upon hearing that Gladwell was ill from alcohol consumption, the committee informed her that she was no longer permitted any strong drink or allowed to have an old stove in her room. Mrs Crofton, applying to enter the Home in 1909, inquired if she could drink stout on the premises. She was given permission, but told that she could have her stout only in her own room, never at the dining table.[113]

Gossip and back talk are hallmarks of the disempowered and marginalized. In the Home for Aged and Infirm Ladies friction did not result in physical action, but rather in dissatisfaction and rumour that fissured through the daily life of the institutional community. The management committee moved swiftly to deal with such situations, always concerned about the public reputation of the institution. In 1910, for example, it was reported that one resident had been telling "falsehoods" about the Home. A delegation of two women from the committee was sent to speak with her.[114] Nine years later a resident was told she would have to leave if she continued to spread reports that were "detrimental to the Home."[115] The 1933 inquiry into Victoria's Maple Rest Nursing Home circled around one story of the owner taking two dollars from a patient and giving him a single banana in return, and another tale of the owner pushing an elderly man down the stairs. Staff and patients repeatedly made reference to these cautionary tales of greed, the abuse of power, and the vulnerability of the elderly.[116]

Residents of old age homes do not fit easily into current analysis of patient advocacy or "grey power." These were not educated, articulate people with connections to the powerful and the knowledge of how to bring about effective change.[117] Looking at post-Second World War English and Welsh institutions for the aged, Peter Townsend found that few residents voiced complaints.[118] Research has shown that when residents of old age homes feel personally insignificant and impotent, they become submissive and retreat to the past.[119] Rebellion, this view suggests, is only for those who can imagine living in a better world. I want to suggest a different view of resistance, a perspective that acknowledges the importance of rebelling itself, quite apart from consequences or the magnitude of the action. I found no instances of organized resistance against institutional regulations or routine, yet the actions and words of the women and men who inhabited B.C.'s homes for the aged give us another picture of the institutionalized aged – a group of people who had no intention of passively accepting their fate.

THE INSTITUTIONAL WORLD: LOSS AND COMFORT

Inevitably, the old age home is a place of loss and finality. The culture of the institutions depicted in this book was indelibly marked by illness and death. The one certainty that most elderly men and women knew when they became residents was that they would only take permanent leave of their new home when they died. Although there were cruel, ageist staff and administrators in these facilities, there were also people who gave from their hearts and had close, caring relationships with residents.

Even early in the twentieth century, when most institutional populations were relatively healthy, administrative records show that inmates regularly fell sick and died. The daily book from the Vancouver Old People's Home charts the departure of ailing men and women to the hospital. Some returned after a short visit, but many died there.[120] In January 1904 the manager of Victoria's Old Men's Home reported that two inmates had entered the Jubilee Hospital during 1903: one had returned in good health but the other had been a patient for more than three months, dying just three days before Christmas.[121] In early February of 1907 Evelyn Jones, a long-time resident of the Home for Aged and Infirm Ladies, was admitted to the hospital. She died there fifteen days later.[122] Inmates would have known that a trip to the hospital might well be their final journey.

Other elderly inmates never went to the hospital, ending their lives in the institution that had become their home. Superintendent Noble at the Provincial Home wrote to the son of a deceased inmate in 1927 to share the circumstances of his father's death. "At breakfast on Tuesday morning," Noble reported, "he [the inmate] said that he had not felt better for a long time and was in good spirits over it and was sitting in his chair in his room when the end came a short time after."[123] In some institutions, including Victoria's Old Men's Home, Allco, and the Provincial Home, there were separate quarters for the sick. But even here, inmates in good health often cared for their ailing roommates, underscoring the omnipresent reminder of what their future held.

This aspect of institutional culture was accentuated by the increase in infirm patients during the 1940s. David Havard remarked in his memoirs of a boyhood spent in Victoria's Old Men's Home that "there always seemed to be somebody dying."[124] Havard's memory is quite accurate: in 1943, when he was a teenager in the Home, thirteen inmates in a population of forty-three men died.[125] On average, one patient died each month. Marpole statistics for the years 1923 to 1938 show a comparatively low death rate: only 50 per cent of the women and men admitted during those years had died by 1938.[126]

But death rates at the Vancouver facility were clearly on the rise, likely reflecting the increase in the number of elderly patients among the institution's population. In 1938 thirty Marpole patients died among a total patient population of 145.[127] Ten years later the statistics for Marpole were little different, but we find that Mount Saint Mary's, which catered to bed cases, reported forty-eight deaths among a population of 101.[128] This is very high compared to what Peter Townsend found in his seminal study of old age homes in England and Wales: studying figures from the same time period, Townsend reported an average death rate of 17 per cent.[129]

We should not assume that all deaths, or even those of close friends, were necessarily emotionally difficult for fellow residents. After all, death was a regular occurrence in these institutions, and an expected event in the lives of the aged. Contemporary studies of old age homes have found that elderly residents typically react with acceptance rather than sadness when another resident dies.[130] Set apart from the familial milieu of grief and mourning that was the norm in the first half of the twentieth century, the institution may not even have been recognized as a legitimate place for strong emotional responses to death.[131] Moreover, as was the case outside residential facilities, death in an institution sometimes had pragmatic consequences that could overshadow emotional reactions. At the Vancouver Old People's Home the death of a fellow inmate might free up a coveted single room. Inmates at the Provincial Home and the Old Men's Home sometimes received clothing or other items that had belonged to former inmates.

Illness and death could, for residents and families, be mediated by the presence of staff who treated the aged with compassionate care, a factor that contemporary gerontologists see as critical in counteracting the dehumanizing effects of institutionalization.[132] Some men and women who administered and worked in homes for the elderly exhibited rare qualities of kindness toward those in their care. The pages of the minute books of the Home for Aged and Infirm Ladies are dotted with notations of thanks from grateful family and friends. In 1913, a daughter wrote thanking the matron and the committee for kindness to her mother, saying that the administration could keep the watch belonging to the deceased woman "for the good of the home."[133] When Miss Robb, long-time matron at the Home, returned from her annual holidays in 1918, "the Old Ladies were quite rejoiced to see her back."[134] One son, writing to the Sister Superior at Mount Saint Mary's in 1958, praised her staff for the attention they gave to the temporal and spiritual needs of their patients. "It always had been my impression," he concluded, "that you do all within your power to give some direction and meaning to the last few declining years of the elderly people residing with you."[135]

Patients at Marpole clearly adored Mary Law, the superintendent, for the special attention she showed them. Law made a point of being accessible to all the patients, taking a personal interest in the particular circumstances of each man and woman in the institution.[136] The fact that Marpole, repeatedly surveyed through 1945 to 1955, always rated high for the care given patients, suggests that the other staff at the institution followed Law's lead.[137] Asked in 1946 if her elderly male boarders thought of her as their daughter, a fifty-eight-year-old Vancouver boarding house operator snorted in reply, "I'm Maw to all of them." Telling a delighted Pierre Berton that she darned the men's socks, turned their collars, and gave them ties or handkerchiefs at their birthdays, "Mother Fowler" stated that "I've got so many children I don't know what to do with them all."[138]

At the Provincial Home and the Old Men's Home two couples, the Nobles and the Havards, provided stable administration during the 1930s and 1940s. Both couples appear to have been tactful and flexible in their treatment of the old men in their care. Harvey noted in 1945 that the administrative staff at Kamloops took a kindly interest in the residents and placed little emphasis on regulation in the institution.[139]

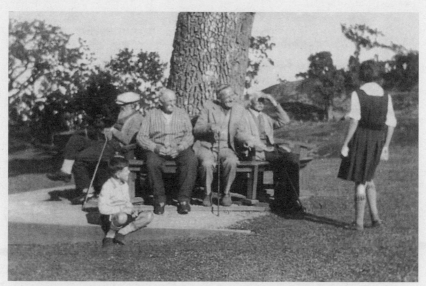

Havard children and inmates of the Old Men's Home, Victoria, 1930s. This informal family snapshot was taken on the bluff behind the home. With the inmates seated around the oak tree and David Havard and his sister at play, it illustrates the close bonds that formed between the residents and local children, especially the offspring of the home manager. The scissor grinder mentioned in the book's section on inmate labour is the bearded man on the far left. (Collection of David Havard)

Here again, the situation at these two B.C. facilities stands in some contrast to other parts of the country where matrons and superintendents were primarily concerned with strict discipline and the results of patient labour.[140] But it is perhaps not surprising that the Nobles and the Havards would have been compassionate toward their aged charges: by the 1940s most inmates would have been in poor or uncertain health and regarded as people who deserved kind and compassionate care. Moreover, a distinct sense of "family" emanates from the Havard memoirs, suggesting elements of the "substitute household" that David Rothman found in the almshouses of colonial America.[141] In a 1928 response to an inquiry about a former resident, Superintendent Havard enclosed a snapshot taken of the man in question and Havard's son with the caption: "Oldest and youngest at the 'Old Mans Home.'"[142]

The Havard family occupied the upstairs superintendent's quarters at the Old Men's Home from 1928 until 1946. David Havard's boyhood recollections contain a number of incidents that demonstrate kindness and compassion toward the old men who shared their home. Mrs Havard allowed one inmate, a former knife and scissors sharpener, to work on her scissors, even though the man's failing eyesight meant that the handles rather than the blades were sharpened. The memoirs testify to the emotional dimensions of such attention: "She [Mrs Havard] endeared herself to H., as she did to many of the old men, through her compassionate nature." Although the roles of husband and wife are interpreted in a gendered light by their son, George Havard's humanity toward the elderly inmates is also clearly revealed. Drunken inmates returning to the Home were not punished but helped to bed. Ill temper was met with patience.[143]

As the case of Mary Law suggests, close ties of affection sometimes developed between administrators and residents. The care and attention that Noble took in arranging the affairs of his deceased bookkeeper in 1937 tell the story of a particularly close relationship. Six months after the man's death, Noble wrote to the dead inmate's sisters that "I missed C. very much at first but have become accustomed to it now." In addition to arranging his friend's funeral, a headstone on his grave, and shipment of his effects back to England, Noble negotiated with the provincial bureaucracy so that the balance of the dead man's estate went to his sisters in England rather than to the provincial government.[144] This rare friendship between two men, an administrator and his inmate-cum-bookkeeper, spoke of commonality of shared administrative tasks: Noble clearly appreciated C.'s professional talents. It also suggests how staff might see the small number of educated or "refined" inmates as different from the mass of unskilled labouring men who entered public institutions.[145]

Yet administrators and staff at institutions for the elderly could also show callous disregard, even cruel behaviour, toward the men and women in their care.[146] There were a handful of complaints at provincial institutions over the years, and hints of poor treatment at private and charitable facilities. Those in charge of B.C.'s old age homes did not judge their elderly charges to be immoral or evil, yet they were sometimes condescending and mean-spirited, and occasionally rough. Investigators into the Maple Rest Nursing Home in 1933 heard that the owner pushed one patient, pulled another's ear, and humiliated one resident who was unable to make her bed neatly.[147] When a resident of the Home for Aged and Infirm Ladies arrived at a committee meeting with a "long list of grievances" in 1914, administrators dismissed her claims as "very irrational" and took the side of the matron instead.[148] But the management did not tolerate cruelty. A nurse was summarily dismissed in 1913 because she was "unkind and unfair" to the residents.[149]

That some caregivers exhibited the tendency to pathologize and trivialize the concerns of the elderly is evident in the professional literature contemporary to the period. The equation of old people with children was common. A woman who worked at the Maple Rest

Nursing Home commented that patients "are not level headed, they are childish."[150] Writing a decade later, an observer noted that "[a]lmost every matron or operator of a boarding home ... conveyed, more or less subtly, his or her sense of the inferiority of the aged." Matrons treated elderly residents like children, she continued, refusing to take their complaints and opinions seriously.[151]

As it is today, death was obviously the one certainty for residents of B.C.'s old age homes in the first half of the twentieth century. However, we cannot know how this fact shaped the emotional contours of institutional life. My research found incidents of both kindness and cruelty by caregivers and strong suggestions that compassionate staff and administrators, like the Havards and Mary Law, brought very real emotional comfort to their charges. One should not ignore, however, the paternalistic attitudes of caregivers toward inmates and patients – be they kind or cruel.

THE WORLD OUTSIDE: FAMILIES AND THE HOME FOR AGED AND INFIRM LADIES

While kin are rarely mentioned in the records of public institutions for B.C.'s old people, family was a vital part of the institutional community of the Home for Aged and Infirm Ladies. In the minute books of the Home, references to family appear on every second page. Indeed, administrators usually juggled two different relationships in regard to each inmate – one with the inmate herself and another with members of her family. Family negotiated on behalf of female kin entering the home and paid for part or all of their keep. The institution was both supportive of the efforts of family to care for aging female kin and prescriptive in their ideas about what families should be doing for their institutionalized elders. Home administrators were also willing to call on family to police the behaviour of troublesome residents. Overall, daughters were most highly involved in the care of their mothers.

Some women entered the Home as independent agents and others as public cases. In a large number of instances, however, sons, daughters, husbands, or brothers were involved in this process, applying for elderly kin to enter the Home and negotiating the terms of payment. Men often approached the Home on behalf of female applicants, committing themselves to monthly remittances. In 1901 the minute books note that Mrs Garneau was entering and her son was to pay fifteen dollars per month for her care. In December 1913 the Reverend Locke wrote to inquire about the possibility of his sister-in-law becoming a resident. Five years later Frank Brett of Hope applied on behalf of his married sister, signing a paper to guarantee payment. Family and Home administrators sometimes worked out payment schemes that incorporated both private and public funding. The minute books for 1905 contain a case of a son paying ten dollars per month for his mother while the provincial government contributed fifteen dollars. The minute books for 1907 note that the son of a Vancouver patient was paying thirteen dollars per month for his mother and the municipal coffers the remaining twelve.[152]

While a pattern of male involvement in administrative matters concerning the institutionalization of female family is evident, the largest single category of kin who made applications or negotiated payment were daughters. Three cases from the 1920s show daughters working to find the best situation for their mothers. In the spring of 1920 Mrs Verchere made an application to get her mother into the Home. The older woman was at the Maple Rest Nursing Home but her daughter could not afford to keep her there any longer. Three months later a woman wrote from Chilliwack about the possibility of placing her mother, currently living with her, in the Home. In 1923 the Home received an application from a Mrs Lancaster whose mother was in hospital but required long-term institutional accommodation.[153]

Small incidences recorded in the Home minute books are poignant testimony to the dedication and love of daughters for their mothers. The attention to small details and comforts is striking. In October 1920 Mrs Coggins asked if her mother might have an extra cup of tea in the afternoon, saying that she would be willing to pay the additional charge. Four years later Mrs Garnet approached Mrs Gould, a member of the Home Committee, to see about getting her mother a lower bed so that her feet could touch the floor when she was sitting up. In this case, kindness was met by kindness. Mrs Gould replied that such a bed would be too low for the nurses to make, but she would have a platform constructed.[154]

Few female residents at the Home for Aged and Infirm Ladies were ever as entirely isolated from their families as the men at the civic home across town. It was not uncommon for women to leave to live with family when circumstances allowed, demonstrating the willingness of many kin to care for aged mothers and sisters, as I suggest in chapter 1. In 1914 Mrs Baird left to live with her daughter. Four years later Mrs Jones departed for her son's home. Another resident left when her soldier son returned after Armistice Day in 1919. This is possibly the same son who had sent Home administrators a letter in 1916 detailing what should be done for his mother in the case of his death. Even long-term residents sometimes departed to live with family.

In 1913 Mrs Garneau, who had been at the home for over a decade, left to make a home with her brother.[155]

Home staff and administrators clearly anticipated that family would continue to play a part in the lives of their aged kin even after they had been institutionalized. This expectation of involvement went beyond merely paying for care, and was policed by administrators on occasion. Negligent children were chastised for not paying due attention to their aged mothers. In 1909, for example, the Home Committee agreed that Mr James be asked "to take his mother out sometimes for a short walk." The 1916 minutes note that "Mrs S's case was considered and the secretary told about her son's promise to come to see her."[156]

Family was often called in to help discipline difficult residents. In 1923 Mrs Napier's daughter was told that her mother must not have brandy in her room and, if the Home rules were not followed, then she would be asked to remove her mother at once. The minute books covering 1947 contain a parallel case. Once again, the daughter of a resident was called in to police her mother's drinking and general behaviour. In 1952 the committee wrote to Mrs Martin's stepson to inform him that his mother was writing letters of complaint to other residents, demanding a room at the front of the building, and had "become a great nuisance." "We would like him," the committee minutes continue in irritable tones, "to come in and see what he can do about it."[157]

While the Home for Aged and Infirm Ladies expected that family should be involved in the lives of their residents, they also supported families by taking in elderly women on a temporary basis. This institutional flexibility allowed caregivers a much needed respite for their work. In 1919, for example, a woman applied to have her mother enter the facility for three months while she went to Banff on holiday.[158] Worn out after caring for her sister for five years, Sally Stanton asked in 1939 if the sick woman could come into the Home for a short period.[159]

Family and institution were interwoven in another manner at the Home for Aged and Infirm Ladies. Over the period covered by the minute books, which span the first half of the twentieth century, I found three clear pairs of spinster sisters resident at the Home. Two sisters entered just before Christmas in 1922, sharing a room and at first paying as private patients.[160] Their money ran out four years later. Another impoverished set of spinster sisters became residents in 1938. The Misses Stewart had only forty-five dollars a month between them for their keep, but the Home administrators did not turn them away.[161]

The economic vulnerability of these four sisters underscores the plight of many childless women in old age.

The continuing involvement of kin in the lives of women at the Home demonstrates that the pattern of family support for older women living outside residential care facilities was duplicated inside the institutional community. Kin took responsibility for finding an institutional home for their elderly female relations, and they often contributed to their keep. Residents sometimes left the institution to live with brothers, sons, or daughters. Family members, especially daughters, continued their work of caring inside the institutional world.

Such family participation was welcomed, even demanded, by Home administrators. Negligent offspring were chastised and children called in to police the behaviour of delinquent residents. Institution and kin, then, existed in a mutually useful relationship, and the institutional culture of the Home for Aged and Infirm Ladies should thus be considered with family in mind. In this pattern of family involvement, I surmise, this Victoria institution heralded the future middle-class old age home where family would be both present and welcome.

THE WORLD OUTSIDE: THE LOCAL COMMUNITY

The old age home and the local community intersected on a number of levels in the first half of the twentieth century. When the inmate population was healthy, the division between residential institution and local community was not as sharp as it is today. Old age homes were not silent, insular places. Instead, able-bodied inmates were a visible presence in the immediate neighbourhood. This interlocking relationship gradually disappeared as increasing numbers of infirm residents and new architectural styles made the institution a place separate from the community, rather than a community institution. I have discussed architecture and the old age home in chapter 2; here I focus on relations between the old age home and the community.

Inmates and patients at old age homes before the 1950s moved easily between institutional community and the local neighbourhood. Residents at the Old Men's Home in Victoria shared their wooden lookout perch with local children, "babysitting" kites tethered to the structure while their young owners ran home for lunch.[162] A 1948 observer noted of one Vancouver boarding house that its elderly male inmates "almost live on the lawn during the summer months," and, of another, that most residents went out the park or down to the beach.[163] In 1953 Miss Hannah, ninety-five-year-old resident of the Home for Aged and Infirm Ladies, reported that she made daily outings into the community in fine weather, sometimes going to the public library to collect books for other residents.[164]

Marpole patients preferred to sit on the sidewalk and observe daily life in the neighbourhood rather than visit the interior garden. Upstairs, bedridden patients coveted places near the windows, which allowed them vistas on the world outside the institution.[165] Windows, architectural theorists of the hospital point out, are extremely important to patients, for they give them something to "supervise."[166] The same is true as well for the elderly who are no longer mobile. In the 1940s, when Isobel Harvey surveyed the institution for the provincial government, the Marpole area was a busy, cohesive neighbourhood, with a lumber mill across the street from the infirmary and an expanding airport on Sea Island. The light industrial base of the area would have had some resonance for the male patients who had worked in primary industries in the province. Harvey noted that "[i]ts neighbours are interested in Marpole and kind to its inhabitants, and no one who has ever seen the infirmary on a fine day will deny that the patients of Marpole are interested in their neighbours."[167]

Life at Allco was entirely divorced from any contact with women, children, and the larger community. As one 1947 news editorial stated, Allco residents were "pushed away out into the wilderness, far from their friends."[168] For many Allco residents life in old age must have been a sad echo of a youth spent in isolated mining and logging camps, unable to hope for the financial resources necessary to establish a home and family. Mount Saint Mary's, designed for bed cases and located on a quiet, non-commercial street, looked out toward the Anglican synod offices and bishop's house on one side and into family homes or apartment buildings on the other.

Communities that contained old age homes were not always happy about having institutional residents abroad in their neighbourhood. One 1938 observer commented on Marpole inmates: "Some Patients ... [who] are able to move about by walking or in wheel chairs sometimes go a considerable distance from the institution and attract unfavourable comment."[169] In 1943, the Mother's Club of the Keary Street United Church in New Westminster protested to their city council about the Salvation Army's plans to build a home for elderly men on the Buchanan Estate at Sapperton.[170] Friction between the institutional community and the local neighbourhood must have been more frequent at facilities that were located in residential areas.

The world of aged single labouring men and the ethos of middle-class familial respectability inevitably clashed on occasion. In order to save both the nearby trees and the sensibilities of passers by, Jane Nixon, the proprietor of the Saanich Health Centre (Royal Oak Private

Hospital), had to police the old men who used an open shed on the premises as a urinal.[171] In 1917 the local police constable complained to the superintendent at the Vancouver Old People's Home regarding the behaviour of one inmate toward young children. The inmate in question denied having done anything untoward.[172] In 1944 Oak Bay parents reported that an inmate at the Old Men's Home was bothering young girls on their way to school, giving them candy and then tripping them up with his stick.[173] "Granny P," one of the most colourful early residents of the Home for Aged and Infirm Ladies, was suspected of stealing a purse on a visit to a local doctor's office in 1903.[174]

Such incidents created tension between the institution and the local community. Administrators, and likely some of the inmates too, were sensitive about attitudes of area residents toward institutional inmates and to the fact that residents might spread disparaging comments about the facility in the local community. George Havard, superintendent of the Old Men's Home in Victoria, wrote of the 1944 incident, "Not only is it unfair to the residents of this district to be subjected to this annoyance, but it also makes it very unpleasant for the many decent old Men that we have here, to be placed in the same category, as this Man."[175]

But in other cases the old age home had a comfortable, even cherished, place in the local community. The Home for Aged and Infirm Ladies was a case in point. Fundraising events were well supported by Victoria residents and extensively covered by the local press. Administrators of the facility used their excellent social and political connections in the city to gain a favoured status for the venerable institution. Residents enjoyed an annual outing to the famed Butchart's Gardens and were personally entertained by Mrs and Mr Butchart themselves on at least one occasion. In 1919 officials from the city police and Government House arranged for the Prince of Wales to interrupt his tour of the city and come inside the building for a visit. Twenty years later residents had special places reserved for them by Alderman Davies to view the royal parade of the King and Queen.[176] The archives of the Home contain a poem titled "To my Neighbours of the Aged Women's Home," in which the author celebrates the different stages of female life, an indication of the personal attachment felt by some in the community to the institution that had been so long at the corner of Rupert and McClure streets.[177]

The Havard memoirs allow us a glimpse of inmates making their own fun, with the indulgent acquiescence of Home staff and members of the community. Havard writes that many of the old men would catch the tram to the nearby "wet" municipality of Esquimalt to indulge themselves: "The street car drivers came to know them all, and made certain the necessary transfer to the Esquimalt tram would see them arrive safely at the watering hole. Some were moderate drinkers, but many overdid, inevitably to return on the last car, again thanks to the compassion and understanding of those B.C. Electric drivers. And when the old fellows poured off at the Home end, my father would be there to get them the rest of the way to bed, with all the attendant problems imaginable. For many, the occasion of the Esquimalt caper was a monthly high point."[178]

Inmates at public facilities received the same charitable attention as residents of the Home for Aged and Infirm Ladies, but never the same affection. In the early years of the institution's existence, members of the public gave used clothing, books, and fruit to the inmates at the Old Men's Home. Victoria's merchants were also generous: in 1893 the Hudson's Bay Company was among those responsible for outfitting the inmates in new woollen drawers.[179] The local branch of the Canadian Legion provided musical entertainment during the 1930s.[180] At Mount Saint Mary's in late 1940s, a regiment of boy scouts and girl guides turned up on Empire Day to take forty wheelchair patients to the parade.[181]

Festive occasions, marked by parties, entertainment, and special treats, also brought children and other people from the larger community inside the institutional world. Christmas and New Year were "two very bright days" for the old men at Victoria's civic home, with presents, good food, and musical performances.[182] Members of the Marpole's Women's Auxiliary always presented each patient with a gift at Christmas.[183] A brownie pack visited the Home for Aged and Infirm Ladies at Christmas, singing carols and distributing candies.[184] At the Vancouver Old People's Home the inmates were treated to special suppers, entertainment by the YWCA and residents of the Children's Home, and a virtual medley of religious services over the holiday season.[185]

The warm weather of the summer months provided opportunities for the residents of old age homes to get outside the walls of the institution, and efforts were made to give the elderly a break from institutional life. In July 1917 fifteen residents from the Vancouver Old People's Home went camping on Bowen Island.[186] The Sisters of Saint Anne took the patients at Mount Saint Mary's for scenic drives around Victoria.[187] The annual garden party for the Marpole residents, arranged by the women of the auxiliary and held at the residence of Mrs Wallace, was a tour de force with pipe bands, swimming displays, and strawberry shortcake.[188]

Some inmates, like the man at the Provincial Home in the 1920s who was active in the church and the Odd Fellows Lodge, continued to be involved with religious and fraternal organizations that had been part of their lives prior to entering the old age home.[189] From 1921 inmates at the Old Men's Home in Victoria were given a weekly allowance for streetcar tickets, allowing them to travel downtown or to other parts of the city.[190]

By the 1950s this pattern of reciprocal interaction between institutional residents and their neighbours had apparently disappeared. I found no more reports of men looking after children's kites or offering them candy. Overall, the old age home was in retreat. It had become a place full of infirm old people whom one could visit, but who ventured out only on special occasions in the care of family or professional caregivers. Brownies, local clergy, and auxiliary volunteers still came into the institution, but they regarded its residents as people who were no longer part of the wider community of neighbourhood and civic society. I imagine that residents of old age homes felt that way themselves.

Despite the reformist ideas of government bureaucrats and medical and social work professionals of the late 1930s and 1940s, established poor law policy and regulations continued to shape the world of the old age home through to the 1960s. Inmates at most institutions were expected to work, to follow regulations, and to be morally upstanding citizens. Many of these practices continued even when other elderly British Columbians were creating lobby groups to fight for better pensions and higher social status and Leonard Marsh and others were crafting Canada's post-Second World War welfare state. B.C.'s aged might have been senior citizens when they were walking the streets of Victoria, but they became poor law inmates once they entered the doors of the old age home.

In public institutions, and in many private and charitable facilities, the presence of a sizeable block of single, working-class men undoubtedly created an institutional character that would have been diametrically opposed to the new ideal being proposed by health and social welfare professionals. Right up into the post-war period, the clientele of public homes in the province was dominated by labouring men. These men brought with them the ethos of male working-class culture. Some used the old age home as part of a seasonal strategy to hold onto an independent life. The continuing dominance of labouring men without families in the institutional populations reinforced the links between destitution and institutionalization. In the years to come, it would mean something only slightly different: if an aged family member was forced to enter a residence, then, conventional wisdom held, it was because the family had somehow failed in its duty.

What did change was the health of the inmate population. Growing numbers of fit elderly men and women were able to use old age pensions to postpone entering an institution. Poor law facilities became nursing homes as the number of frail and sickly elderly in their care increased. Public institutions for the elderly in the province had always been places of destitution, but the cultural context was now defined by illness and death rather than by punishment and need. In a sense, the old age home evolved toward being a "total institution" as inmates were less able to move in and out as they chose.

It is evident that residents of old age homes suffered from a loss of independence. Resistance to institutional authority took many forms, both passive and actively rebellious. Again, we might suppose that, as the population became less healthy, overt resistance and patient agency became less common. Yet while these facilities essentially served as places for the aged poor to die, we can also see that some inhabitants found a sense of community and small pockets of pleasure in their institutional home. Overall, these were more generous places than the bleak workhouses that housed the aged poor in other parts of Canada.

5 Community Care or Institutional Care? Early Welfare State Strategies

"Care in the community" and "sheltered accommodation" are the buzzwords of geriatric care at the turn of the twenty-first century.[1] In British Columbia and elsewhere across Canada, innovative community programs have given people unprecedented opportunities to remain in their own homes as they grow older and infirm.[2] Regardless of which place on the political spectrum they come from, both current professional thinking and state policy are strongly supportive of old people remaining outside the old age home.

Those who formulate and implement community living programs tend to present their work as modern and unprecedented. Today's gerontologists, however, should conceptualize these programs within a longer historical continuum. Community care for the aged in fact fits into an older pattern of out-relief and boarding out that has often existed as part of poor law and welfare state provision. The historical use of hospitals as welfare institutions for old people is another important theme in this regard. While no one would be so foolish as to suggest that the past repeats itself, bringing the longer view into policy analysis can help us understand the historical provenance of contemporary health and welfare policy.[3] Policy, like institutions (the most tangible manifestation of policy formation), bears the indisputable and indelible imprint of the ideology and time that give birth to it. Moreover, as the research that underpins this chapter confirms, there are important continuities in terms of policy practices and concerns. Historical analysis can facilitate a breadth of discussion and discourse by drawing the past into contemporary studies.

In this chapter I explore a fascinating experiment in community care that took place in British Columbia during the inter-war years. In 1937 the provincial Liberal government, headed by Premier T.D. Pattullo, brought in the Hospital Clearances program, a plan to find non-institutional solutions to the dilemma posed by elderly and infirm long-term hospital patients. The clearances scheme was no ad hoc response to the social and economic horrors of the Depression, but a structured program based on a careful study of hospital patients in the province. Aged or chronically ill people who did not require constant medical attention were to be taken out of hospitals and boarded with local people in their home communities.

The Welfare Institutions Licensing Board was the other major policy initiative concerning the elderly taken by the Pattullo government. Scandalous revelations about the abuse and manipulation of the vulnerable aged led to the 1938 Welfare Institutions Licensing Act, and the new legislation brought the licensing board into being to monitor residential facilities caring for indigent men, women, and children. Old age homes and their clients were drawn closely into the net of an increasingly regulatory provincial state that was dominated by professional bureaucrats.

The goal of de-institutionalizing aged people too infirm and impoverished to live independently was not met. A decade after legislation created the Hospital Clearances program, the political and professional will to seek viable community care options had dissipated. Instead, under successive Coalition and Social Credit governments, a network of private, public, and charitable old age homes developed. Private hospitals took the majority of elderly public patients, replicating the hospital model at a reduced cost for the public purse. Funding for the small number of public institutions for the aged in the province evolved from a poor law to a welfare state model. The provincial state took on a substantial role as regulator of private and charitable old age homes, encouraging development through cost-sharing and grant schemes.

B.C.'s pioneering community care program was part of a provincial shift toward centralization and professionalization in public health and social welfare policy initiated by George Weir, the provincial secretary in the Pattullo government.[4] While Ken Moffatt's recent history of Canadian social work demonstates that social work thought of this era was more diversified than coherent, my research points to some critical commonalities among the range of new policies that were developed in the western province during the Pattullo years.[5] Scientific methods, medical specialization, an emphasis on professionalism, and financial backing from the Rockefeller Foundation were all hallmarks of B.C.'s reform program. Hospital finances were restructured and

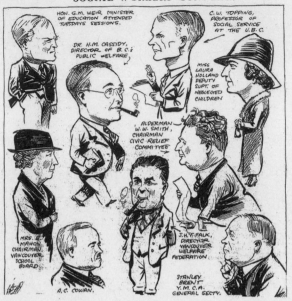

Vancouver *Province* editorial cartoon, 1934. Drawn by B.C. cartoonist Jack Boothe when the provincial Liberals came to power under T.D. Pattullo, this image depicts the cluster of social welfare bureaucrats, activists, and academics that worked together to transform welfare services in the province during the Depression era. Several key individuals in the move to reform residential care for the aged are depicted in this cartoon: Laura Holland, Harry Cassidy, and George Weir. C.W. Topping spearheaded professional training for social workers at the University of British Columbia, providing staff for the new provincial Welfare Field Service.

regularized, community medicine was rationalized, specialized medical divisions were created to deal with venereal disease, tuberculosis, and vital statistics, and a provincial laboratory system was established.[6]

Pattullo's Liberals, in power from 1933 to 1941, brought the notion of corporate government to the western province, believing that state and society was best run by "experts." Trained professionals would mediate the rights and demands of varied interest groups.[7] In B.C., the work of the Welfare Institutions Licensing Board and of the Hospital Clearance staff served to highlight a specific (and needy) population of elderly people at the same historical moment that gerontology was emerging as a speciality in Britain and the United States.[8] Welfare professionals within the state bureaucracy, rather than medical practitioners or scientific researchers, emerged as B.C.'s first specialists in geriatric care. Most of these new experts were women. While today policy rarely bears the stamp of a single individual, this was not the case in the early development of the welfare state in Canada: programs of the 1930s and 1940s were often formulated over a short time span by a small group of civil servants. For this reason I pay close attention to the ideological beliefs, career aspirations, and professional agendas of the health and social welfare bureaucrats who formulated and administered geriatric policy in B.C.[9]

B.C.'s Hospital Clearances program and the Welfare Institutions Licensing Board should thus also be understood in a wider framework, beyond the context of Weir and Pattullo's provincial reforms. The cluster of age-specific health and social welfare policy initatives that came out of B.C. during the 1930s and 1940s were part of a vast social project of twentieth-century western society that set the elderly aside and began establishing a structured "timetable" for the last decades of the life cycle. Jill Quadagno and William Graebner rightly situate the impetus for this change within the confines of the state.[10] W. Andrew Achenbaum, Carole Haber, and Thomas Cole emphasize the role played by the medical and social work professions.[11] In this chapter I bring all these parties into analytical play.

This chapter considers why the clearances program was unsuccessful and assesses the system that developed in its place. I begin by describing the clearances program and the Welfare Institutions Licensing Board as they were first conceptualized, and chronicling their evolution during the 1940s. I then analyse the failure of the goal of community care and the emergence of gerontology as an area of health and welfare specialization in B.C. The chapter's final section looks at the network of residential facilities for elderly people that had been put into place by the post-war period, with emphasis on how successive provincial governments dealt with the issue of old age and institutionalization. The analysis in this section extends into the late 1950s and early 1960s to show how the old age home fit into federal hospital policy during the post-World War Two period.

HOSPITAL CLEARANCES AND THE WELFARE INSTITUTIONS LICENSING BOARD: THE ORIGINS OF WELFARE STATE POLICY FOR THE INSTITUTIONALIZED AGED

Aged men and women emerged as primary clients of the Hospital Clearances program and the Welfare Institutions Licensing Board. This gave the provincial welfare state a much larger role in the regulation of the lives of elderly people who were in need of sheltered accommodation.

Ten years after the board was established an observer commented that no other province in the country had such a broad provision for the inspection and regulation of these facilities.[12] Nor were there schemes similar to the Hospital Clearances program in other parts of Canada at this time. Ontario, for example, did not begin a similar program until the late 1950s.[13] In Britain attention was focused on long-stay patients only after hospitals were brought under the umbrella of the National Health Service in 1948.[14] Those who originally formulated the B.C. scheme were proud of the innovative nature of the program.[15]

B.C.'s early entry into this field of geriatric care was shaped by a complex blend of professional personalities and agendas, economic expediency, and the bureaucratic requirements of the emerging welfare state. Change began to take place in 1937, four years after the Liberals had come into power. Before this, many elderly who were ill and indigent were placed in local hospitals, a process that went on with the co-operation of families, physicians, and local authorities.[16] But the modern twentieth-century hospital, designed to care for patients with acute conditions, and increasingly drawn toward science and technology, had no place for such patients.[17] As Charles Rosenberg points out, the medical agenda of the hospital superseded its earlier function as a welfare institution.[18] What was different in B.C. was the systematic nature of the clearances program and the key role played by the state.

Before the Liberals, the provincial government paid hospital grants on the basis of occupied beds. This meant that municipalities and individuals were the beneficiaries of provincial coffers, particularly if patients had monthly pension cheques to sign over to the hospital. The incoming Liberals criticized this arrangement, citing Victoria's Jubilee Hospital as a particular offender.[19] Thus, a strong point of principle regarding responsibility and jurisdiction underpinned hospital clearances: the local municipality was meant to care for these people, so they should be returned to the community to which they belonged.

Dr Gregoire Amyot was appointed adviser on hospital services and assistant provincial health officer in 1936 with a mandate to survey existing hospital services and formulate a new hospital policy. A medical doctor with a diploma in public health from the University of Toronto, Amyot had also spent a formative professional period with the Michigan State Health Department and the Rockefeller Foundation. In 1936, when Amyot was asked to undertake the survey of B.C.'s hospitals that became the basis for the Hospital Clearances program, he had been director of the pioneering North Vancouver Health Unit for a decade.[20] Amyot's subsequent report made no direct reference to the fact that most chronic patients were old people. This is not surprising because Amyot was not looking for the elderly *per se*; in his professional paradigm the aged were not yet a specific category. Indeed, if Amyot "saw" these older patients in an age-specific way, it would have been through the Rockefeller lens as used up, irreparable machines that did not belong in the hospital, a modern centre of technology and scientific medicine.[21]

Amyot did not work alone on the hospital survey, the first of its kind in the province. He had "discovered" his colleague, Percy Ward, in North Vancouver, where Ward was manager of the North Vancouver General Hospital, instigating an eight-hour work day for nurses and standardizing record-keeping and bookkeeping. Ward went on to become provincial inspector of hospitals, a position that he held until his retirement after the Second World War.[22] Although Ward lacked Amyot's professional training, both men believed that standardized systems and central administrative control would correct problems with hospital accounting and long-stay patients.

The two men found that public patients remained in hospitals much longer than private patients. In the twenty-two hospitals studied, there were 108 patients who had been in hospital for more than 300 days. Amyot and Ward identified most of these patients as "social-problem cases," people who did not need to be in hospital.[23] Indeed, their use of the term "social-problem" itself suggested that they viewed these people as the property of social workers rather than medical personnel. The province government responded to these findings with the Hospital Clearances program, announced in the fall of 1937. In January 1938 the government added teeth to the new policy, cutting provincial funding to patients who stayed longer than 300 days. This forced hospitals like the Royal Jubilee in Victoria, which had been caring for forty-one chronic patients, to take action. The Jubilee Hospital terminated their contract with the city to care for indigent patients in February. By March alternative arrangements had been made for eighteen of the Jubilee patients.[24]

Provincial bureaucrats believed that the clearances program made good economic sense. In a speech given to senior provincial health and welfare staff in January 1937, Amyot argued that hospitals would save 10 per cent of their annual operating budgets if they could reduce the stay of this group of patients.[25] Writing four years after the program was implemented, Percy Ward commented that the 108 hospital clearance cases that Amyot and he had identified in 1936 had cost the province approximately $28,000 yearly in hospital grants. Public patients who required long-term care could be cared for much more cheaply in facilities designed specifically for that purpose.[26] The subtext of these statistics and plans was that municipalities, not the province, should be paying for these patients in some other setting.

Amyot's professional involvement ended once the survey was complete. In his mind, the chronically ill patients had now vacated the public hospital and the way was clear for the expansion of scientific medicine. Thus, over the first years of its existence, B.C.'s Hospital Clearances program was shaped by New Liberal beliefs in rational planning and social work methodology rather than by medical science.[27] Harry Morris Cassidy, the University of Toronto academic hired in 1934 as B.C.'s first director of social welfare, was an important figure behind the new program. Born in B.C., Cassidy took his first degree at the University of British Columbia, and then went on to obtain a Ph.D. in economics at the Brookings Institute in the United States.[28] Cassidy emphasized both the humanitarian values of improved public welfare services and the importance of employing scientific methods and efficient planning.[29] His deep and lifelong faith in the social work profession is evident in the broad role that he assigned to it in the new hospital clearances scheme.

Laura Holland was another pivotal person in this burgeoning provincial administrative apparatus. Trained in social work at Simmons College in Boston, Holland worked in Montreal, Toronto, and northern Ontario before coming west to B.C. in 1927 to reorganize the Vancouver Children's Aid Society.[30] Holland was regarded by Cassidy and other progressives in B.C.'s fledgling social policy circle as a trusted and proficient colleague, well able to take on challenging new roles. In 1935, already working within the provincial ranks as superintendent of neglected children, Holland was placed in charge of the incipient Welfare Field Service. As the first supervisor of the new service, Holland was responsible for transforming a nucleus of five former mothers' pensions visitors into a professional group of twenty-five university-trained social workers.

Working together to develop the new clearances program, Holland, Cassidy, and Ward soon found that it was the indigent elderly who were occupying costly hospital beds.[31] But even in the first stages, when the composition of their clientele had not yet become apparent, all three individuals favoured a social work approach to the clearances. In 1937 the provincial welfare fieldworkers added to their already impressive array of tasks the job of transferring elderly patients from local hospitals to the homes of relatives or to foster homes.[32] This cadre of professional social workers thus became the first gatekeepers for the Hospital Clearances program, working on the front lines to implement new policy directives in the community.

This element of welfare professionalism in the clearances program had significant implications. Cassidy and Holland looked for workers who were young, sympathetic to their "underprivileged" clients, able to work well with others, and adept at spreading the gospel of preventive social work in local communities.[33] They were to employ standardized methods of investigation and reporting.[34] The work of placing elderly men and women in local homes or institutions was not easy. In Revelstoke in early 1939, we find a beleaguered fieldworker placating an elderly male client who, she believed, had "numerous persecutory ideas," while also trying to impress upon local medical personnel the need to gather specific information and follow regularized procedures.[35]

There was a strong commitment within the provincial bureaucracy to the principle that social workers in the field should be trained professionals.[36] Known as Cassidy's "university girls," the women were mostly social workers trained in the University of British Columbia's new social work program. This educational background, quite different than what James Struthers found among Ontario social workers of the period, ensured that the social case work method so highly prized by Cassidy, Holland, and Cassidy's successor, George Davidson, became an integral part of how elderly clients were treated.[37] The use of professional personnel and of detailed medical and social case reports enhanced the power of expert over personal testimony.

Historians of old age see strong links between the marginalization of the elderly in modern society (the modernization thesis) and growth of "expert" opinion about the aged.[38] The case of B.C.'s clearances program shows how a client group – in this case the elderly – can emerge from policy, rather than policy being created with a specific clientele in mind. Elderly people have been "hidden," not just in public institutions, but in public policy formation. At the same time, B.C.'s health and social work professionals helped to create the category of "elderly" as a client group beset by personal, social, and medical problems.

In my mind, the interaction between client and welfare fieldworker points to the resurgence of a new variety of poor law paternalism within the modern welfare state. The large numbers of single aging male clients in the program meant that female social workers took on the role of surrogate mothers, sisters, and daughters. In these guises welfare fieldworkers, like their professional colleagues inside the old age home, made professional judgments with far-reaching consequences. They were interested in assessing not the morality of their elderly clients but their personality and their physical and mental capabilities. All these personal characteristics were interpreted through the lens of their professional culture. Reflecting the political bias of their new employers, the professional values of these men and women were steeped in New Liberalism. Their focus on environmental explanations for social problems, rather than broader social and economic concerns, was characteristic of the profession during the 1930s and 1940s: in Canada and the United States social workers showed a new concern with professionalism and a desire to see social problems in relation to the individual, not society.[39]

In the early years of the program, when the social work ethic held sway, there appear to have been greater efforts made to take an individualistic approach to clients. Whenever possible, elderly people were placed in local homes rather than distant institutions. Re-admission to another public facility was meant to be a last resort, with the goal being to place patients in inexpensive local boarding homes.[40] Vancouver and Victoria's social service departments were given funding to operate their own hospital clearance schemes. In 1937 the City of Vancouver received $3,000 to set up a program.[41] The following year Vancouver was given a grant of $1,500 and the City of Victoria $1,200. Welfare fieldworkers outside the two major urban centres added to their other tasks of investigating relief, mother's allowance, child welfare, and tuberculosis cases the job of working in conjunction with local hospitals and doctors to place chronic patients in foster homes or with friends or relatives.[42]

B.C.'s Hospital Clearances program was shaped by professional agendas and bureaucratic expediency. In contrast, the impetus for the Welfare Institutions Licensing Board initially came from outside the government. Two scandals concerning the plight of the institutionalized elderly caught the attention of B.C. in 1937. The first was a sad tale of petty cruelty and manipulation of aged inmates at Homes for the Friendless in Burnaby and Summerland. One couple had been refused $2.50 spending money from Home administrators although they turned their pensions and savings over to the institution. Other residents were intimidated and fearful of physical injury if they made complaints.[43]

But the exposé of the Homes for the Friendless paled beside the sinister activities of the Collins family. Vancouver detectives Fish and Hoare found that Violet and William Collins had operated a series of homes for elderly people and unmarried mothers in various parts of the city, making use of numerous aliases. The Collinses often moved into the house owned by the old man or woman for whom they were caring, and continued to live there after the death of their patient. There was an unusually high death rate among mothers, babies, and elderly residents in facilities run by the couple.[44]

The Collins case placed institutional care for the aged onto the political agenda at a moment at which the provincial welfare state was posed for dynamic expansion. The Liberal government moved swiftly in response to these two cases, setting up first one and then another commission of investigation. The first provincial commission, conducted by

H.I. Bird in 1937, looked specifically at the two Homes for the Friendless. The 1938 commission was broader in scope, investigating a total
of ninety-one facilities, including boarding homes for indigents, nursing
and convalescent homes, children's homes, and private hospitals.
Licensing, fire and health inspections, medical and nursing care given,
rates charged, records kept, and the living conditions of patients were
all studied.[45]

These two commissions, and the shocking cases that had prompted
their investigations, were a benchmark in the history of old age homes
in the province. Bird recommended that legislation be created to provide for the registration and licensing of institutions like the Homes
for the Friendless, and that these facilities be inspected on a regular
basis. The 1938 commission report, which followed the enactment of
the Welfare Institutions Licensing Act, argued that there was a need
for even tighter regulation and for standardized inspection and licensing.[46] In the two reports the institutionalized elderly were constructed
as a specific category of people who were both defenceless and deserving. Often without family to monitor the care they were receiving,
liable to have their savings taken by unscrupulous caregivers, the aged
men and women in these institutions were clearly in need of vigilant
care by the state.[47]

The Welfare Institutions Licensing Act came into effect on 1 April
1938.[48] The act covered public and private institutions that housed
children under age twelve, pregnant single women, unemployed adults
receiving financial aid, and "aged, infirm, or physically handicapped
adults on public assistance."[49] This legislation brought private and
public charitable institutions and boarding homes that took public
charges under the regulatory arm of the state. Pre-existing laws had
governed private hospitals and nursing homes, as was the case elsewhere in Canada, but there was no regulation of boarding homes that
took in public indigents, and only one hospital inspector to do the work
required for the whole province. As was the case with the Hospital
Clearances program, the number of elderly clients that emerged was
an unanticipated development. As Laura Holland, donning another
bureaucratic hat as the first inspector of welfare institutions, noted in
her 1942 annual report, the majority of the work performed by the
inspectors related to homes for the aged.[50]

Although the Welfare Institutions Licensing Act was a direct result
of the findings of the 1937 Bird Commission, there was a close link
between the board and the Hospital Clearances program. The fact that
many residents of welfare institutions were hospital clearance cases,
the second commissioner argued in 1938, meant that they were "entitled to the same measure of protection as are patients in recognised

hospitals and no one would deny that the latter are entitled to the best in way of attention and protection."[51] Under the clearance scheme, the province sought to decrease its financial responsibility for this group of infirm and indigent aged and move them out of public institutions. However, the provincial state then became morally obliged to ensure that clearance patients were placed in reputable facilities where care was of a good standard. By taking on a regulatory role, the provincial state would ensure that it continued to perform its public and moral duty for this vulnerable sector of the populace.

Laura Holland was instrumental in shaping the work and structure of the Welfare Institutions Licensing Board in its first years of operation. The administrative wing of the new bureaucratic structure was a board of five people, including the provincial superintendent of child welfare and a member of the provincial board of health. The other three board members were provincial civil servants. Under the terms of the act, the board had the power to formulate regulations governing welfare institutions in the province without legislative or ministerial approval. This structure, which was undoubtedly the result of Holland's formulations, vested considerable power within the bureaucracy and meant that Holland and her colleagues were able to impose their professional agendas on the work of the board. As one observer noted, "[i]t [the act] enables the individuals who administer it to enforce a good standard now and work towards enforcement of a higher standard in the future, without limiting their power in any way to put into practice new and more progressive regulations." Four office staff were responsible for supervising and inspecting proposed or existing welfare institutions.[52]

The board's annual reports show that the fledgling department was both vigilant and proactive: over time a clear agenda emerged to push institutions for the aged toward new ideals of care. Holland perceived her role as educational rather than punitive. Using an approach that reflected her considerable administrative savvy and social work training, Holland usually gave institutions time to correct shortcomings and comply with the standards set out by the act, rather than take immediate disciplinary action. Thus, although an impressive total of thirty-one organized institutions and boarding homes for the aged and handicapped were inspected during the first year of Holland's work, only four licences were granted. The majority of those that remained were set aside for further investigation.[53]

Holland was not the only high-ranking female bureaucrat who dealt with institutions for the aged during the late 1930s and 1940s. Following Holland's career path, two other women became central figures in the development of hospital clearances and welfare inspections in B.C. Edith Pringle, a registered nurse, was put in charge of the Hospital

Clearances program in 1937. Her mandate was to plan and promote medical social work and clearance schemes in hospitals throughout the province. Five years later she was appointed deputy inspector of welfare institutions as part of departmental restructuring.[54] When Percy Ward retired in 1948 Pringle became provincial inspector of hospitals, the first woman to hold that post.[55]

Pringle's earlier professional work had included hospital administration and nursing education. Her hospital clearance experience broadened her expertise to include social work practice and made her one of B.C.'s first specialists in the care of the elderly. By 1944 she was an active member of an advisory committee on the care of the dependent aged.[56] A year later the Fort George Chapter of the Registered Nurses Association of British Columbia enthusiastically reported that Pringle had talked to them about community support for the elderly.[57] Pringle's colleague Edna Page joined the welfare institutions inspection staff as a social worker in June 1942, and was promoted to deputy inspector in January 1943. In 1942, the provincial inspection of welfare institutions was brought within the administrative confines of the provincial office of the inspector of hospitals and became the responsibility of these two women.[58]

The Hospital Clearances program and the Welfare Institutions Licensing Board proved to be a fertile meeting ground for the professional categorization of the aged and the growth of the welfare state bureaucracy. A noteworthy feature of both the program and the board in their early years was the significant presence of professional women at all levels of the bureaucracy. This may have been because women were seen as the appropriate bureaucratic guardians of the vulnerable, signifying a link between the emerging professional welfare state and older maternal feminist ideas. A closer ideological link may have existed specifically between female professionals and the elderly. Women were, after all, a significant presence among the slim ranks of American social gerontologists from the 1930s onward.[59] In B.C. during the same period, many of the students in the provincial university's master's program in social work who did research on aging were also women. As researchers and practitioners, social gerontology was clearly a field where a woman could make her mark. Health and social welfare bureaucrats may have been trying to meet the needs of their elderly clients, but they were also creating gendered professional enclaves within the state system by advancing the programs for which they were responsible.[60]

As I make clear, the Hospital Clearances program was not specifically intended as a policy for geriatric patients. Rather, like the Welfare Institutions Licensing Board, it evolved into a scheme that primarily

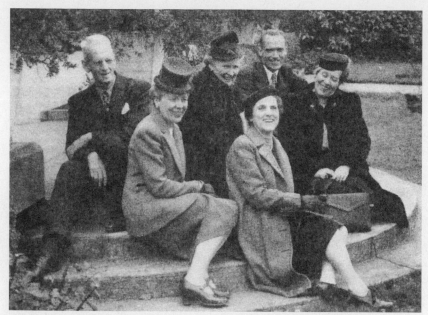

Percy Ward's hospital inspection staff, 1946. This group of provincial bureaucrats was responsible for creating and maintaining a standardized system of inspection for non-medical residential facilities for the aged after the Welfare Inspections Licensing Board was created in 1938. Edna Page, assistant inspector of institutions, and Edith Pringle, a registered nurse and inspector of hospitals and institutions, both seated to the right of the photograph, ran the welfare institutions inspection scheme, becoming two of B.C.'s first geriatric specialists. Percy Ward, seated on the left, assisted Gregoire Amyot in his 1936 study of the use of acute care hospital beds by chronic patients and was a key figure in the Hospital Clearances program that followed. (National Library, Ottawa)

served old people, rather than being designed with that purpose in mind. Thus, what we see in B.C. was an organic development of a client group of elderly men and women. The parallel growth of a cluster of female experts in gerontology was another unplanned result of the new schemes. What was more intentional was the pivotal role played by the social work profession in this process. The professional agendas of Cassidy and Holland, two of the key people responsible for designing and implementing the new programs, favoured social workers and the social work method. We should not forget, however, that the Hospital Clearances program began as reform with an economic purpose: the needs and concerns of the elderly men and women who became clients of the new bureaucracy were thus secondary to the fiscal and administrative requirements of the state.

ASSESSING THE ABANDONMENT
OF COMMUNITY CARE: PATIENTS,
PROFESSIONALISM, AND POLITICS

The concept of community care for aged public patients in British Columbia during the late 1930s proved to be a short-term experiment. By 1939, only two years after the clearances program had begun, it was clear that the institutional solution would dominate. This trend continued. During the 1940s provincial bureaucrats put into place administrative procedures that favoured professionalism and large institutions over local programs and smaller facilities. As reports from Victoria and elsewhere show, the majority of clients simply ended up in another institution.

Over time, social workers and bureaucrats picked institutions over local boarding houses and private homes because they found that it was the fastest, most efficient solution to a growing problem. For example, Florence Mutrie, Victoria's assistant relief officer, began by using a variety of solutions to deal with hospital clearance cases. In the spring of 1938 she handled a caseload of forty-four individuals, arranging for ten to board in the homes of local women and two to return home. The rest went to other institutions. Six men were placed in the municipal Old Men's Home, the same number of women went to the local Home for Aged and Infirm Ladies and two men applied to the Provincial Infirmary. Eleven men and women were admitted to local private hospitals.[61] Thus, even at the program's outset, institutional care dominated. Indeed, administrators at the Home for Aged and Infirm Ladies noted at their May 1938 annual meeting that all their vacancies had been taken by clearance patients.[62]

By 1939 Victoria's relief department was apparently no longer attempting to place convalescent cases from local hospitals in the community and had instead established a nursing home program. Mutrie moved clearance cases to convalescent homes, the Home for Aged and Infirm Ladies, the city's own Old Men's Home, and likely the Chinese Hospital. In 1939 forty-seven such cases were being cared for in private facilities. In 1940 the Relief Committee reported that the City Welfare Department had placed a total of 139 patients since the beginning of the clearances program and were currently making use of two convalescent homes and eight nursing homes and private hospitals. The following year the city's health and welfare committee noted that there were forty-nine city patients being cared for under its nursing home program. Thus, without a consciously stated change of policy, the practice in Victoria evolved toward a complete dependence on the institution.[63]

There are a handful of reasons for this evolution. First, the growing numbers of clearance cases meant that there was less time for individualized solutions and more pressure on social workers to place clients in institutions. Second, the concept of community-based care for the elderly was never supported by the enhanced community structures that have been key to successful projects today.[64] Third, bureaucrats overtook social workers in rank within the provincial bureaucracy, making economic and administrative efficiency a priority. And finally, subsequent governments were less interested in innovative health and social welfare programs than Pattullo's Liberals had been. The history of the Hospital Clearances program suppports Linda Gordon's belief that most welfare policies are the product of conflict and compromise and should be conceptualized as such.[65] The clear vision of Holland, Amyot, and Cassidy in 1938 had grown muddled and increasingly bureaucratic by 1945.

Reading Amyot and Ward's survey in 1937, Holland and Cassidy thought that they were looking at a single block of patients that needed to be shifted from the hospital into the community. But the number of clearance cases requiring transfer out of hospitals did not diminish as predicted. On the contrary, the demand for places always exceeded what was available, and the patient backlog grew longer each year. In 1939, the most successful year of the program, 86 per cent of the total cases handled were dealt with. Yet in no other year between 1938 and 1948 do the statistics show such success. During the early years of the Second World War approximately 67 per cent of cases were placed. In 1943 only 53 per cent of cases were placed, and by 1945 this figure had dropped to 36 per cent. In 1945 the annual report noted that the number of hospital clearance cases who had died before they could be moved from the hospital had doubled.[66]

The lack of local resources was another contributing factor. With ever-growing lists of elderly people needing placement, there were neither sufficient numbers of kin to take in their elders nor people willing to board elderly men and women. A characteristic community caregiver for an elderly clearances patient would probably have matched the profile of people who took in public boarders a decade later: a housewife with an extra room and a desire to earn some money in her own home. In the 1930s, however, women and families were still under-represented in many of B.C.'s resource-based communities, meaning that there was not always a large pool of caregivers on which administrators could draw.

Chapter 1 details ad hoc community support systems for old people, but university-educated social workers from outside the settlement may not have been well placed to utilize these resources for hospital

Figure 3
Hospital clearances, 1938–1948

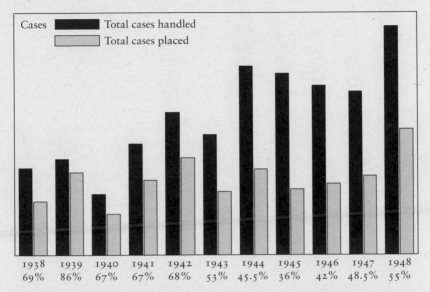

| | Cases | ■ Total cases handled |
| | | ▢ Total cases placed |

	1938	1939	1940	1941	1942	1943	1944	1945	1946	1947	1948
	69%	86%	67%	67%	68%	53%	45.5%	36%	42%	48.5%	55%

Source: Province of British Columbia, Department of the Provincial Secretary, *Hospital Statistics and the Administration of the Hospital Act, 1948.* Victoria: King's Printer, 1949.

clearance cases. Community discussion about home care for the aged did not begin to emerge among social workers and public health officials in Vancouver and other parts of Canada until the mid 1940s. Laura Holland and her colleagues were formulating policy nearly a decade earlier, in the political vacuum of the Depression. The general mobility in B.C.'s resource-based economy probably also had an impact on the willingness of women to take elderly hospital patients into their homes. Products of the large transient male workforce discussed in chapter 1, many older hospital patients would have been strangers to potential caregivers and less welcome in their homes.

Finally, the strong orientation toward professionalism within the hospital clearance bureaucracy was likely another important factor in the shift toward an institutional solution. B.C.'s welfare professionals of the 1930s and 1940s never expressed a strong commitment to placing elderly people in local boarding houses or back into their homes. Community care is essentially anti-professional in nature, giving agency to the needs and wishes of the client over the professional and the state. I see the institution and the clinic, rather than the broader community, as the key sites of professional development during this period.

Ageism within the social work and nursing professions also served to foster negative attitudes toward the elderly and deny them agency. As described in chapter 3, professional attitudes embodied two prevailing concepts of the elderly – the aged as dysfunctional and the aged as victim. While many social workers were kind to their elderly clients, there was clearly a darker professional perspective that saw older kin as an unhealthy element in the family. Contemporary social work discourse about elderly people is rife with comments that exemplify this view.[67] Negative stereotypes of the aged also rationalized their continued institutionalization. If elderly men or women could not be healthy members of their own extended families, why should they be placed in other peoples' homes? And conversely, if the aged were as vulnerable as the 1937 and 1938 commissions of inquiry had found, then they were best off in an institution.

Structural changes within the provincial welfare administration were probably another factor in the abandonment of community care for B.C.'s institutionalized aged. The 1942 administration reorganization that brought together the work of Pringle and Page also amalgamated the welfare field branch with the provincial unemployment relief and old age pensions offices. This merger brought male relief investigators with very different professional attitudes into the hospital clearance field at the local level. The business backgrounds of the new workers, many of whom were placed in supervisory positions over the incumbent field staff, clashed with the co-operative approach and social work methods of their female colleagues.[68] These "unemployment relief men" were schooled, not in the Social Work Department at the University of British Columbia, but in the milieu of Depression relief programs.[69] It is possible that these former relief workers would have had little regard for the time-consuming work involved in placing old people in local boarding establishments or finding a way for them to return to their own homes.

Another reason for the adoption of the efficient institutional option lies in the checkered history of provincial politics. The Liberals under T.D. Pattullo, the government responsible for the initial legislation, ran the province from 1933. Pattullo's more radical health and social welfare agenda was blunted by the October 1941 election, which brought the defeat of George Weir. Two months later Pattullo's own party deserted him.

The Coalition government, a partnership of Liberals and Conservatives intent on keeping the left-wing Co-operative Commonwealth Federation out of government, was in power from 1941 to 1952. There was considerable tension within the Coalition over health and social welfare issues. As might be expected, the Liberal members of the coalition government wanted to continue to expand social services; the Conservative members opposed social reform.[70] This split was reflected in the lack of firm direction in policy concerning institutional provision for B.C.'s aged, and the 1940s were a time of ad hoc solutions rather than clear policy directions.[71] In terms of the Hospital Clearances program and the Welfare Institutions Licensing Board, this impasse meant that no new policy initiatives emerged during the Coalition period. Old people were simply not on the political agenda. Moreover, it is likely that provincial bureaucrats like Amyot, Holland, and Ward were able to take advantage of the vacuum left by the lack of political will, moving policy in the direction they considered best.

The right-wing Social Credit Party, which pushed the bickering Coalition government out of power in June 1952, followed a similar policy line regarding old age homes to that held by their Conservative predecessors. But by this point the political climate had shifted: concerns about "senior citizens" were evident in political and public discourse.[72] Grassroots Social Credit party membership was definitely sympathetic toward the aged who suffered financial hardship, and believed that old age homes were an important issue.[73] Yet while W.A.C. Bennett, the new premier, shared this belief in social programs, he held firm to the view that new health and social welfare expenditure must be funded from growth in the industrial and economic sectors.[74] In the Social Credit equation, therefore, welfare services must follow economic prosperity rather than social need. Moreover, Bennett's government continued to argue that the indigent aged were a municipal charge, rather than a provincial responsibility.

Thus, the demise of the hospital clearance scheme as it was first envisioned by Amyot, Cassidy, Holland, and Ward was the result of several different factors. The number of elderly people requiring residential care was overwhelming and seemingly never-ending. This meant that a system that counted on the work of lay women and local community, in a region where both were in relatively short supply, was clearly unworkable. Community care can only work, obviously, where community exists, and in western culture that means women. Certainly, there was also stagnation and a lack of ongoing innovation at the political level. It is unlikely that successive governments would have initiated or supported a substantive community care program. But perhaps most importantly, this system neither served the interests nor met the ideological ideals of the health and welfare professionals who had moved into positions of power. The bureaucracy was the place where dynamic processes were at work, and it therefore held the most power in determining policy and program direction.

THE STATE, CAPITAL, AND CHARITY: THE POST-WAR PICTURE

Instead of a viable community care program for the de-institutionalized elderly, what evolved in British Columbia over the 1940s was a network of private, charitable, and state institutions that took clearances cases and other elderly infirm. This network was the direct result of the dynamic put into motion by the hospital clearances. State funding had a substantial impact on the kind of institutional care that evolved in B.C.: as was the case in other countries, the state had the power to stimulate or repress markets in care facilities for the aged. In Australia, for example, private nursing home accommodation mushroomed once state funding was secured.[75] American historians argue that the Social Security Act of 1935 and the 1960s Medicare and Medicaid programs fostered the growth of private old age homes.[76] Britain's private care facilities for the elderly withered under the post-war welfare state and thrived under Margaret Thatcher.[77] In B.C., the provincial state set up funding schemes to encourage the growth of municipal and charitable old age homes. Ultimately, however, both municipalities and the province became highly reliant on private care facilities for elderly people.

A "mixed economy" of provision thus emerged in B.C., with a strong dependence by the state on private hospitals and an infusion of funds from various levels of government.[78] This blend of state, voluntary, and private involvement was similar to that which Jane Lewis and others have found in other times and places, but in this case the layered nature of the Canadian state (federal, provincial, and municipal) was an added factor. Old age homes thus moved within the policy confines of the post-war welfare state: administratively, they came under the policy umbrella of hospitals and away from welfare policy *per se.*

Inevitably, there was tension between municipal and provincial governments over the question of who was responsible for the care of the indigent elderly. Municipal authorities were often unhappy with the hospital clearance scheme because it cost them more to house patients in private facilities than in public hospitals. In 1940, for instance, a patient's care in a nursing or convalescent home cost the City of Victoria one dollar per day, with the provincial government making no contribution. But if the same patient remained in an acute care hospital bed it cost the city only seventy cents each day, with the government contributing approximately the same amount. In an effort to pressure the province to provide funding for nursing home clearance cases and enlarge the Provincial Infirmary system, the Vancouver City

Social Service Department stopped participating in the program between 1942 and 1948. The City of Victoria also attempted to persuade the provincial government to share the cost of maintaining hospital cases in nursing and convalescent homes.[79]

Bowing to the fiscal realities of residential care for the elderly, the Coalition government began making regular payments to municipalities during the 1940s to help them cover the cost of housing the elderly on state assistance. From 1941 the province paid up to 80 per cent of the cost of keeping chronic patients in boarding homes and welfare institutions, with municipalities paying the remaining 20 per cent, and in 1948 entered into another 80/20 fiscal arrangement, this time to cover the cost of nursing home care.[80] Yet throughout the decade the provincial administration steadfastly maintained that clearance patients were the responsibility of the local community, not the provincial state. The Coalition government was willing to make regular support payments for individual cases, but it held back from committing itself to the ongoing maintenance of publicly funded old age homes.

The province also tried to encourage municipalities, religious groups, and non-profit societies to build public institutions for the infirm elderly. In 1947 the Coalition government initiated a program that paid a portion of the construction costs of non-profit old age homes. With this program, and in paying for individual patients, the Coalition government was able to show that it was protecting the vulnerable aged and providing for their needs. Like the Sisters of Saint Ann, who had been commissioned to provide care for the elderly at Mount Saint Mary's in 1941, religious and non-profit groups were definitely considered suitable caregivers by the general public. This last point was important, for by the 1940s the public was becoming interested in the question of institutional care for the aged.

The Victoria Nursing Home, built by a non-profit society just as the Second World War ended, set a precedent for the 1947 provincial construction program. The new facility was established with joint provincial/municipal funding four years before the cost-sharing program started. The City of Victoria provided the $25,000 needed to purchase the building and property, while the provincial government granted $7,500 to supply furnishings for the new forty-four-bed facility. Funding from the city was contingent on a number of conditions, one of which was that 60 per cent of the beds in the new home were reserved for city indigent cases.[81]

Bennett's government initially continued to follow the same policies as their predecessors, acting as a watchdog on private and charitable old age homes, funding the construction of municipal and non-profit facilities for the elderly, and making transfer payments to municipal governments for their indigent elderly. The major policy initiative of the Social Credit government concerning geriatric residential accommodation was the Chronic Treatment program. Announced with fanfare in 1956 by Eric Martin, minister of Health, the new program called for the establishment of chronic hospitals. Patients for these facilities would be limited to those with treatable chronic conditions. Both the Social Credit government and the federal authorities, who were negotiating with B.C. politicians to fund chronic hospitals, were anxious that funding be funnelled to patients whose health would benefit from treatment.[82]

The Chronic Treatment program was neither a political nor an administrative success. Because the federal government required that patients receiving funding be "treatable," most elderly residents at the Victoria Nursing Home, Mount Saint Mary's, and similar facilities were not covered.[83] Two years after the new program had been announced, civil servant Lloyd Detwiller wrote to his superior, Donald Cox, commissioner of the B.C. Hospital Insurance Service, that "[v]ery little has been done to implement this program on the basis as outlined in the Minister's proposal."[84]

Yet this fledgling program was more important than the slow pace of its development suggests. The new policy was a tacit recognition that municipalities could not cover the entire cost of either building or running facilities for the elderly and chronically ill. Payment for the program was meant to come from individual patients, municipalities, and the province: the province and municipalities were each to pay seventy cents per diem, and the patient was to be charged one dollar for each day of care. Perhaps most significantly, the new coverage was designed to fit within the National Health Care program when it became operational.[85]

Thus, while the Chronic Treatment program itself had minimal impact, it was a bridge to the universal extended care and nursing home programs of the next decade. In spite of repeated federal assurances to the contrary, the general public continued to believe that coverage would extend to nursing homes.[86] In 1953 a column on nursing homes appeared on the women's page of the Victoria Times, provoking a "flood of letters" in response.[87] Nearly all the writers spoke of the need for greater government involvement in establishing good care facilities for the elderly. Provincial bureaucrats filed these articles in government correspondence, demonstrating that provincial bureaucrats and politicians were sensitive to the public concern about housing for the elderly.

The expansion of welfare state provision for old people meant that institutions now received funding from several levels of government.

A combination of federal, provincial, and municipal funding resulted in complex fiscal structures. Public patients at Mount Saint Mary's, for example, were housed in facilities built with provincial funds. Their keep was paid from municipal, provincial or federal coffers. In provincial, and municipal institutions, pension cheques from the federal state became a substantial part of patient revenue.

This interweaving of funding meant that older public institutions like the Old Men's Home in Victoria and the Provincial Home for Aged Men now based their fiscal operations on a combination of traditional poorhouse financing and welfare state economics. In Victoria, for example, improvements to the Old Men's Home were still financed by the inmates' "entertainment fund," based on funds signed over to the city by incoming residents. The construction costs of a new lavatory in 1942 and 1943 repairs to the Home were paid for in this fashion.[88]

By the 1940s, revenue from old age pensions was a significant source of funds for public facilities like the Old Men's Home. In the United States, the 1935 Federal Social Security Act, which denied funds to residents of public institutions, helped push the hated almshouse into historical memory.[89] In Canada, pensioners in state old age homes were compelled to turn over their pensions to administrators, thereby ensuring the ongoing existence of these institutions.[90] In effect, the federal government was subsidizing institutional care for elderly patients in these facilities. Institutional records show that administrators in provincial, municipal, and charitable homes were active in securing pensions for residents.

Pension income therefore became part of the economy of older institutions like the Home for Aged and Infirm Ladies, the Old Men's Home, and the Saanich Health Centre. This was clearly the case at Victoria's Old Men's Home, where pension income covered approximately half of the facility's operational costs from the late 1930s. In 1937, for instance, Superintendent George Havard reported that net receipts from pensions and assignments totalled $5,000 while estimated costs for the year came to $10,000. This left the city with a bill of $5,800 for the maintenance of thirty-two men for the year ($181.25 per inmate). When a man was hired at sixty dollars a month to assist the superintendent in 1942, the funds came from the increased pension income that was entering the coffers of the Home.[91]

Private hospitals had been used by the state for elderly indigents before the Hospital Clearances program, but after the clearances scheme came into operation the numbers of public cases funnelled into this care sector increased dramatically. With a chronic shortage of beds in public institutions for the infirm aged, and few charitable facilities in the province, social workers and hospital authorities had no option but to utilize private hospitals and boarding houses to care for hospital clearance cases. By 1946 municipal and provincial authorities were noting that the shortage of beds for elderly patients was allowing private nursing homes to raise their rates substantially.[92]

Increased demand for accommodation for public patients meant that the growth in size and number of private facilities was accelerated. As noted in chapter 2, the business of providing residential care for the aged became more profitable and more tightly regulated by the state. Private hospitals evolved from small institutions run by independent women into corporate business interests closely linked to the expanding welfare state. Within the institutional economy of the private hospital, the money brought in by state patients was significant. By the mid 1950s the state was paying for 73 per cent of all patients in private hospitals in British Columbia.[93] A 1956 snapshot of thirty-six private hospitals in Greater Vancouver demonstrates the monetary significance of elderly public patients. Five hospitals relied solely on welfare clients. In nine other facilities public patients comprised more than 80 per cent of the clientele. Only two institutions reported that less than 50 per cent of their patients were funded by the state and just six took no welfare patients at all.[94]

The provincial government was never comfortable with its high reliance on private hospital care. This was the Achilles heel of the clearances system, and civil servants and politicians knew it well. Bureaucrats themselves criticized the system that they had helped establish. Laura Holland, for example, was arguing as early as 1944 that the use of profit-making institutions for the aged was only a short-term solution.[95] A year before the Chronic Treatment program was announced, Donald Cox, provincial hospital insurance commissioner, bluntly informed Eric Martin, provincial minister of Health, that elderly pensioners simply could not afford to pay the cost of institutional care for an ailing spouse and still cover their own living expenses.[96] There was concern, as well, that the operators of private nursing homes would create monopolies of care, forcing the province to pay substantial fees for elderly public patients.[97] It was his opinion, Cox wrote to Martin in 1956, that the government would eventually have to take financial responsibility for nursing home care.[98]

Politicians became increasingly aware of the high level of distrust with which the general public viewed private nursing homes, and of the fact that many old people were unable to pay for a lengthy stay in a private hospital. One woman told of her efforts to care for a dying father in a 1955 letter to Premier Bennett. She asked that modern nursing homes be built to "help bridge the gap of old age between their failing hours and the grave."[99] Gerald Pelton, founder of the

Old-Age Pensioners' Organization, wrote to Martin, minister of Health, in the same year, arguing that "the crying need of the aged today is an assurance that when they become helpless, they will have care and comfort, free from the fear of still further reduction in their living conditions when their funds are exhausted."[100] By 1961, with men and women over the age of sixty-five comprising 10.2 per cent of the province's population, the Social Credit government was wise to take such concerns seriously.[101]

The 1957 federal Hospital Insurance and Diagnostic Services Act specifically excluded nursing homes, yet it served to place the concept of a new social minimum in hospital care, provided to all on equal terms, on the post-war policy agenda. Responding to pressure from the public and from their own civil servants, provincial politicians became increasingly persuaded that the state would have to pay for nursing home care. In 1964 Martin wrote to Lt Col J.W. Duncan, secretary of the Vancouver and District Council of Churches. He detailed his government's work to support community efforts to encourage nursing home and rehabilitation care, and finished his letter by stating his hope that the federal government would soon amend the hospital insurance program to cover nursing homes.[102] At the July 1963 Conference of Health Ministers, and through correspondence in 1964, Martin pressured Judy LaMarsh, federal minister of Health and Welfare, to reinterpret the kind of care provided by nursing homes and bring them within the scope of the 1957 Act.[103]

By the end of the 1950s, of the established triad of residential care institutions for elderly British Columbians – state, private and charitable – private hospitals dominated, providing care for aged clearance patients in a setting that resembled the institutions that they had just left, for a fraction of the cost that had previously been paid by the province. As was the case in Britain with the National Health Service in 1948, and in the United States with the Social Security Act of 1935, changes in provision for the aged in one sector of government brought evolution in another arena of jurisdiction as well. Federal old age pensions, for example, became a core part of the institutional economy of B.C.'s public homes for the elderly. The Hospital Clearance scheme was the initial impetus for whole system of state funding and institutional provision.

It is significant that the last phase of growth in this institutional sector took place in an era of dynamic developments in federal hospital policy. Policy makers began to think of homes for the aged as medical institutions rather than welfare facilities, in part, no doubt, because the clearance program had made such significant use of private hospitals for elderly people. The passage of the federal Hospital Insurance and Diagnostic Services Act ensured that debate concerning institutional care for the aged was based on the assumption, at least at the provincial level, that there would eventually be a place for this level of coverage under the federal program. Public sentiment, management support, and, finally, political will, all favoured this solution.

Early hospital clearance initiatives attempted to place elderly patients in homes in their local communities, but in the long run, the large numbers requiring placement, the lack of a community base, and bureaucratic demand for efficiency all contributed to the dominance of a more simple institutional solution. The failure of the Hospital Clearances program to achieve its original policy objective thus cemented an ongoing dependency on the old age homes.

There are a number of other reasons why this early and fascinating community care experiment was doomed to failure. First, the clearances program was never a community initiative. It was simply an attempt by provincial civil servants and politicians to make local communities, through their municipal governments, take responsibility for their medical indigents. Second, with the exception of some limited fieldwork done by local social workers to find women willing to take old people into their homes, there was no effort made to build local community structures to support the policy. Indeed, such an enterprise would have been out of keeping with professional ethics of the period. Third, this was a program devised by policy makers, who were not entirely sure who their clientele was, and who were mostly concerned with saving money. Again, this only makes sense in the middle of the Great Depression.

Overall, the trend was toward greater state responsibility for institutionalized elderly in the province. The findings of the Bird Commission and the Welfare Institutions and Nursing Homes Commission in the late 1930s underscored the fact that the dependent elderly could be manipulated and abused in unregulated accommodation. Because the aged were seen as defenceless, the state was obliged to protect and care for them. The extension of state intervention through the provincial regulation of welfare institutions meant that provincial bureaucrats became directly responsible for many more aged clients than they had previously. Civil servants like Laura Holland and Edith Pringle became the province's first geriatric specialists.

A network of institutions for old people was established in B.C., combining state involvement with private enterprise and charity. Although the concerns of the aged themselves were not incorporated into policy decisions, this was a mutually beneficial situation for the other parties involved. Federal old age pension income provided a financial base for public and philanthropic old age homes. Municipalities and charitable groups received provincial money to build homes for the elderly. Private nursing homes expanded, relying on a steady income from public patients. And the provincial state was able to transfer direct responsibility for some of the impoverished aged under its care to municipal, charitable, and private concerns. By maintaining vigilance over homes for the aged through the Provincial Office of Hospital Inspection and the Welfare Institutions Licensing Board, such an approach was legitimized.

Taking the long view, one can see in the growth of state involvement in the regulation and provision of old age homes the historical genesis of current residential programs for elderly British Columbians. The presence of profit-making business interests in the field made it inevitable that the public would become uncomfortable and anxious with private ownership in this service sector. During the 1940s and 1950s, the media and the general public accepted that the growing need for accommodation for the aged would integrate state funding, private capital, and charity. By the 1960s, this compromise was no longer considered acceptable. The aged, now more numerous and considered to be a particularly vulnerable and deserving group, merited finer treatment by a compassionate society. Increasingly, the state was seen as the most appropriate provider of residential care for the aged; this group was simply too vulnerable to be left to the uncertainties of capitalist enterprise. Calls for state-run residential care facilities for the dependant aged eventually resulted in the implementation of the provincial Extended Care and Nursing Home programs in the mid 1960s.

Conclusion

Our understanding of the development of the old age home in Canada must take into account the historical moment at which the institution came into being in different regions of the country. Institutions, odd and metamorphic creatures that they are, bear forever the stamp of the era in which they were constructed and the purpose for which they were created. The old age home in British Columbia stands apart from patterns of institutional evolution in other parts of Canada. The pace of non-aboriginal settlement was different in the west, where residential facilities for the elderly were established later than in eastern and central regions of the country. The founders of old age homes in B.C. acknowledged that the aged were predominant among society's needy and that institutions specifically for elderly indigents were most appropriate, and so public and charitable old age homes were established as such, rather than evolving from houses of industry.

The old age home in B.C. was different in a second respect. The scattered nature of settlement in much of B.C. forced the provincial government to take a larger, more active role, both in providing and policing residential facilities for the aged. During the 1890s the Provincial Home for Old Men and Victoria's Old Men's Home were established. Yet overall, municipal activity in this sector was very slow – just five years after Victoria's municipal administration had agreed to open a home for elderly men, it refused to sponsor a home for impoverished old women. Vancouver, the province's major urban centre from the 1890s, did not build a municipal home for the aged until 1915. Charitable efforts for the elderly were similarly limited. Until the 1940s, when provincial funding stimulated growth in this sector, there were only two long-established charitable homes for the elderly in B.C.: the Home for Aged and Infirm Ladies and the Chinese Hospital, both in Victoria.

In charting institutional developments from the 1890s to the 1950s, this study reveals another interesting pattern – the use of local hospital beds on a consistent and long-term basis by indigent elderly in the period before the Second World War. This relates in part to the lack of municipal services and the surplus of single men in the province, but it also underscores the importance of looking for old people in a variety of institutional settings. Before the elderly were regarded as a unique social group, they were not always identified as a specific category, readily apparent to the historian of old age. This point also applies to health and social welfare policy. Elderly indigents were one of the primary recipients of the provincial Indigent Fund, a precursor to old age and mothers' pensions. The history of the Hospital Clearances program and the Welfare Institutions Licensing Board also demonstrates we have to look for old age in policy that does not immediately reveal itself as directed at the aged. Over time, these programs led to the significant expansion of provincial and municipal state involvement in the provision, funding, and regulation of institutional facilities for the aged.

Demographically, the western province has always had a distinctive population of elders. From the early period of non-native settlement in the nineteenth century until well into the twentieth century, white and asian old men in B.C. outnumbered their female contemporaries. Many of these single men had worked in B.C.'s resource-based industries. Often without family and savings, they were particularly vulnerable as they aged. By the 1940s these men had been joined by Prairie retirees wanting to spend the final phase of their lives in a more temperate locale, but it is the first group that comprised the worthy "pioneers" for whom B.C.'s first old age homes were built.

The question of just how much responsibility the state should take for providing and regulating institutional care for people like these single old men has been negotiated and renegotiated over time. The British historian of old age and the welfare state David Thomson suggests that it is best to view provision for the elderly as a broad, ever-shifting continuum, with the state or community at one end and the family at the other.[1] He argues persuasively for the view that the English family was never really seen as responsible for its elders and that state provision has been relatively generous, even in the harshest decades of the New Poor Law administration.[2] In B.C. the issue of responsibility for the aged was resolved in families and local communities in a number of ways. Marriage, home ownership, and helpful children were crucial variables for old people trying to hold on to an independent lifestyle. A range of commitment from offspring is evident, but, overall, most children were willing to provide some support for their aged parents, especially for their mothers. I found many instances of rural communities taking considerable responsibility for the elderly, raising money on their behalf or petitioning the government for monetary assistance. In urban centres "community" was more narrowly defined by race, class, and neighbourhood. This book demonstrates conclusively the agency of elderly men and women in their quest for independence, and the importance of old age pensions in this regard.

I have approached the question of responsibility for the care of the aged from different perspectives throughout this book. In Canada, a distinctive feature of old age policy is the way in which the different levels of the state negotiate with each other regarding assistance for the elderly. Most B.C. municipalities did not open old age homes until after the Second World War, holding fast to the idea that they were not obliged to. The provincial state took a much larger share of responsibility for the dependent aged over the period covered by this volume, establishing a Provincial Home for Old Men in the late nineteenth century and setting up a Provincial Infirmary system for the infirm indigent elderly. Apart from a handful of First Nations residents at the Home for Incurables, the federal government assumed no direct responsibility for the institutionalized elderly in the province.

This picture changed from the beginning of the 1940s, however, as the province retreated from the direct provision of residential accommodation for the aged and municipal and federal levels of government became significant players. The province tried to situate itself as a watchdog over residential care facilities. By the middle of the 1950s the province had expanded its regulatory powers over old age homes and set up funding structures to encourage municipal governments and philanthropic groups to establish old age homes. Its use of private care facilities for public patients resulted in substantial growth in this sector. Municipalities all over the province transformed existing physical plants into old age homes and built new structures. The federal government, which had provided indirect funding to institutions through old age pensions since 1927, was poised on the edge of the picture, ready to move directly into the area of health provision with the 1957 Hospital Insurance and Diagnostics Act.

This book therefore bridges the progression of the old age home from a poor law facility to a medical institution under the umbrella of the welfare state. I see this shift as important yet little understood, for residential care institutions are not commonly thought of as the building blocks of the modern welfare state. Theorists of the welfare state and social policy for the aged see old age policy as a central plank in the construction of the welfare state and a useful avenue to wider discussion of the growth and nature of the modern welfare state,[3] but for the most part, they have passed over the old age home. Those who do look at twentieth-century care facilities emphasize the heritage of the workhouse in the modern old age home, thereby obscuring the important ways in which institutions for the elderly have served the agenda of the professional welfare state. The historical development of old age homes in B.C., however, demonstrates strong links between the development of a network of private, public, and charitable nursing homes and the growth of a professional welfare state.

The old age home underwent significant evolution from the late nineteenth century to the middle of the twentieth century. In the nineteenth century old people without money were placed with other indigents in municipal workhouses or, if they were more fortunate, in one of the new philanthropic old age homes being founded across North America. These were not medical institutions but rather places that emphasized morality, charity, thrift, and punishment.

By midway through the twentieth century, when this study concludes, there had been considerable change. The wider use of old age pensions, which allowed people on limited budgets a greater bid at independent living in their last decades, meant that the populations of old age homes became increasingly elderly and infirm. With higher rates of infirm elderly, old age homes moved from being welfare institutions to being health care institutions.

Class and professionalism intersected in the evolution of the old age home into a medical institution. This was a parallel process to what American medical historian Paul Starr calls the "moral assimilation" of the hospital, where a social organization constructed for the poor is transformed into a respectable, middle-class institution.[4] The modern nursing home, a middle-class institution with close links to the welfare state, had emerged. Ideally, this revisioned old age home was to be staffed by medical and social work professionals and run on a medical model. The theme of "home," as envisioned by middle-class volunteers and professionals, was emphasized in new décor and an emphasis on sociability between residents.

These changes suggest a new, re-visioned old age home, a place where the promise of a compassionate post-war Canadian society would unfold. But the old age home has in fact become a world apart: it is an institution that has turned inward. Residents no longer come and go, leaving independently to work or visit friends and family. Informal interaction between residents and local people, like David Havard's tales of lunchtime comradery between children and inmates on the bluff behind Victoria's Old Men's Home, is now rare. I want to take you now to visit Greenwoods, a continuing care facility constructed on Saltspring Island in the early 1970s. Built adjacent to the local hospital and outside the commercial and social hub of the town of Ganges, the design groups the residents' rooms around an inner courtyard: the vista is to the inside rather than the ouside. Although a more recent decision to place a pre-school daycare facility within its grounds suggests a positive step toward community integration, Ganges, with its bookstores, market, park, and cafes, is a half mile distant – too far for any resident to reach independently for shopping or coffee with a friend from outside Greenwoods.

Yet while places like Greenwoods have ceased to be community institutions, neither have they been entirely successful in establishing a new status as medical facilities. People do not go to these places to be healed, after all. Elderly women and men only leave Greenwoods, if they leave alive, to go into the extended care ward of the neighbouring hospital. There is little place for medical technology in the old age home, or indeed in the "hospital" accommodation of extended care facilities. Staffed by women, the second sex, the old age home demonstrates how female professionalism, middle-class domestic architecture, and an elderly clientele served to undercut an institution striving for medical legitimacy.[5] Residential care facilities for the aged thus remained second-rate medical institutions, much lower in the institutional hierarchy than general hospitals and psychiatric centres.

And perhaps most perniciously, the ghost of the poorhouse has lingered on into the second half of the twentieth century. It lingered first in the old public poorhouses with vast wards and drab dining rooms, in the cramped urban boarding houses, in the ostentatious discarded dwellings of the rich and powerful, and then it crept into the bright "modern" municipal homes. It has lingered among the people who live in the old age home, the lonely logger with a bad back, and the impoverished Victoria spinster. It has lingered in the practices of old age home, the regimentation and the rules to be followed. And it has lingered in social attitudes toward residential care facilities, in the fear of institutionalization that underpins the strategies of many old people. Perhaps this is why the house of old remains a place that gives us so little comfort.

Notes

ABBREVIATIONS

BCA   British Columbia Archives
BCLL   British Columbia Ligislative Library
NA   National Archives of Canada
OB-DHM   Oak Bay Municipality, Clerk's Office, David Havard, "Memoirs"
RMC   Rose Manor Collection
SMA   Saanich Municipal Archives
SP   *Sessional Papers, British Columbia*
SSAA   Sisters of Saint Ann Archives
UTA   University of Toronto Archives
VANCA   Vancouver City Archives
VCA   Victoria City Archives
VCA-CR   Victoria City Archives – Committee Reports

INTRODUCTION

1 Atwood, *morning in the burned house: new poems*, 85–7.
2 Laurence, *The Stone Angel*.
3 Rogers, "First Christmas Away From Home."
4 MacPherson, Dr J., interview.
5 Katz, "Poorhouses and the Origins of the Public Old Age Home."
6 Himmelfarb, *The Idea of Poverty*; Finlayson, *Citizen, State and Social Welfare*; Crowther, *The Workhouse System*; Katz, *Poverty and Policy*.

7 Struthers, *The Limits of Affluence*.
8 Rule 12 of the Home stated "No person admitted to the Provincial Home shall, so long as he is an inmate of the same, be entitled to vote at any provincial Election." Rules and Regulations for the Government of the Provincial Home, 25 July 1895, BCA, GR 496, Box 12, File 1.
9 In an earlier period, both Britain and the U.S. established systems of local poorhouses which housed needy elderly along with the handicapped, the mentally ill, single mothers, and children. For an analysis of the development of poorhouses in the United States see Katz, "Poorhouses and the Origins of the Public Old Age Home," and Haber, *Beyond Sixty-Five*, 82–107. For Britain, see Thomson, "Workhouse to Nursing Home." In the Canadian context, the best summary of this institutional activity is in Snell, *The Citizen's Wage*, ch. 2.
10 Forbes et al., *Institutionalization of the Elderly in Canada*, 5–6.
11 Cook, "'A Quiet Place ... to Die,'" 26–7; Stewart, "The Elderly Poor," 217; Morton, "Old Women and Their Place," 11.
12 Haber, *Beyond Sixty-Five*, 83–4; Katz, "Poorhouses and the Origins of the Public Old Age Home," 110–40; Crowther, *The Workhouse System*, 89–90; Morton, "Old Women and Their Place," 11.
13 Crowther, *The Workhouse System*, 270 and Katz, "Poorhouses and the Origins of the public Old Age Home."
14 Stewart, "The Elderly Poor," 222.
15 Morton, "Old Women and Their Place," 11.
16 Perkin, *The Rise of Professional Society*; Skocpol, *Protecting Soldiers and Mothers*; Gordon, "The New Feminist Scholarship"; Struthers, *The Limits of Affluence*.
17 The best analysis I have read concerning ageism is in Peace et al., *Re-evaluating Residential Care*, 54.
18 Hareven, "Life-Course Transitions and Kin Assistance"; Anderson, "The Impact on the Family Relationships."
19 For a thoughtful discussion of the use of patient names set in the context of mental health institutions, see Reaume, "Portraits of People with Mental Disorders."
20 Snell, *The Citizen's Wage*.
21 The concept of independence is a critical component of the way in which historians of old age have approached the study of elderly men and women. See Laslett, "The Traditional English Family," 115–64, and Hareven, "The Last Stage," 13–27.
22 For a discussion of this approach see Phillipson, *Capitalism and the Construction of Old Age,* and Smith, "The Structured Dependence of the Elderly."
23 Thomson, "Workhouse to Nursing Home," 43–69.

24 Because Canada Census did not look at institutional populations during the period that I study, it is not possible to calculate precise numbers of elderly residents. I used available census material and provincial statistics for private hospitals and welfare institutions. My figures are approximations because the age of residents was not noted.

25 The 1931 federal census found 308 people over sixty-five years of age in charitable and benevolent institutions in B.C. See *Canada Census*, 1931, vol. 9, table 9, 281. There were 290 beds in private hospitals (excluding maternity hospitals) in the province in 1934. See Province of British Columbia, *Hospital Service and Costs*, 1934, 11.

26 BCA, GR 496, Box 49, File 5, Province of British Columbia, Department of the Provincial Secretary, *Report Regarding the Administration of the Welfare Institutions Act*, 1941, table 2, 12, and *The Administration of the 'Hospital Act'*, 1941, 1942, Table 7, 23.

27 Province of British Columbia, Department of Health and Welfare, *Report on Hospital Statistics*, 1957, 1958, 44–5.

28 In comparison to the growing number of institutions caring for the aged, the number of institutions for children requiring total care and for pregnant women remained constant, at eleven and three respectively, over the years studied. *SP*, 1951, vol. 3, 1953, W-100.

29 BCA, GR 678, Box 10, File 25, Edith Pringle, "The Need for Chronic Disease Hospitals," 1953.

30 Stewart, "The Elderly Poor"; Snell, *The Citizen's Wage*; Struthers, *The Limits of Affluence*; Montigny, *Foisted upon the Government?*

31 Janeway, *Powers of the Weak*.

32 Townsend, *The Last Refuge*.

33 For a fuller discussion of links between the economy, demography, and health care of B.C. see Davies, "Mapping 'Region' in Canadian Medical History."

34 Rudy, *For Such a Time as This*, and Guildford, "Closing the Mansions of Woe."

35 Clough, *Old Age Homes*, 4–8.

36 Peace et al. make this point brillantly in *Re-evaluating Residential Care*, 4–5.

CHAPTER ONE

1 As described in n21 to the Introduction, historians of old age have stressed the importance of independence to elderly men and women. See Laslett, "The Traditional English Family," 115–64, and Hareven, "The Last Stage," 13–27.

2 Anderson, "The Impact on the Family Relationships," 36–59.

3 This was true in Ontario for the late nineteenth and early twentieth centuries. Struthers, *The Limits of Affluence*, 52–3.

4 The most useful discussion of the concept of "underclass" in welfare history is Katz, *Poverty and Policy*.

5 New Zealand was also a male-dominated settler society. In 1871 there were 705 women to every 1,000 men, with a much larger imbalance in frontier areas. As late as 1914 there were nearly as many bachelors as married men. Phillips, *A Man's Country*, 7–11.

6 Historians have emphasized the transient nature of B.C. society and the small number of non-aboriginal women during this period. See, for example, Barman, *The West Beyond the West*, 89–90 and 148–9. Martin Grainger describes the coastal logging life in *Woodsmen of the West*, a wonderful memoir of male culture in early twentieth-century B.C.

7 Statistics compiled from the *Canada Census*, 1901–1961.

8 Ward, "Population Growth in Western Canada," 169–170.

9 This analysis of the lives of single male labourers in B.C. is based on the following sources: Harris, "Industry and the Good Life," 194–218; Mouat, *Roaring Days*, especially ch. 6; Wynn, "The Rise of Vancouver," 111–12, and Anderson, "Sharks and Red Herrings," 43–84. For memories of the male world of logging and mining camps see Knight, *A Very Ordinary Life*, 195, 202–4, and Knight, *Along the No. 20 Line*, 111–16. Danysk shows how, in contrast to much of B.C., rural prairie communities came to be organized around the family and the family farm. "A Bachelor's Paradise," 156.

10 Knight, *Along the No. 20 Line*, 55–8. Knight's story of the working life of Ebe Koeppen includes an excellent description of a coastal logging operation in the 1940s, 111–16.

11 Cole Harris provides a sensitive discussion of how the economics of mining life and the geographical isolation of mining communities made marriage an impossible dream for most men. "Industry and the Good Life," 203–5.

12 Johnston, "Native People, Settlers and Sojourners, 1871–1916," 192.

13 Con et al., *From China to Canada*, 5.

14 Canada census data cited in Lai, "From Self-segregation to Integration," 65.

15 Johnston, "Native People, Settlers and Sojourners, 1871–1916," 192.

16 Anderson, "The Impact on the Family Relationships," 46. Townsend also found this in his study of institutions for the elderly in England and Wales. *The Last Refuge*, 290–1. Looking at the period 1877–1907, Stewart found that the aged population at the Wellington County House of Industry in Ontario was 82 per cent men. "The Elderly Poor," 224. Twenty-four of twenty-seven inmates at Ottawa's Protestant

Home for the Aged in 1887 were men. Cook, "'A Quiet Place ...
to Die,'" 29. See also Katz, *Poverty and Policy*, 111, and Crowther,
The Workhouse System, 234.

17 Tennant, "Elderly Indigents and Old Men's Homes," 3–20.

18 BCA, GR 131, Box 1, Vol. 1. The following inmate numbers were
selected for analysis, spanning the admission years 1895–1965: 1–99,
300–99, 600–99, 900–99, 1,200–99, 1,500–99, 1,800–99.

19 BCLL, Harvey, "Study of Chronic Diseases."

20 BCA, GR 131, Box 3, Envelope Mc, N.M. to A. Noble, 4 January 1925.

21 VANCA, Series 452, Box 106F1, File 1, List of Persons in the Home,
1907–1911.

22 Parr, *The Gender of Breadwinners*, 188, notes the difference between
married and single men in this respect. See also Morton, *Ideal Surroundings*, 36–7.

23 Grainger, *Woodsmen of the West*; Harney, "Men Without Women," 216.

24 This point is made about the Hungarian bachelor immigrants by Kosa,
Land of Choice, 28 cited in Harney, "Men Without Women," 230n72.
This attitude toward single old labouring men was held by social work-
ers and government bureaucrats in B.C. during the 1930s and 1940s.
Davies, "Old Age in British Columbia," 64–5.

25 BCA, GR 289, Box 7, File 2, Government Agent, Vernon to P. Walker,
16 June 1925 and Government Agent, Vernon to P. Walker, 29 May 1925.

26 BCA, GR 496, Box 17, File 2, New Notes, vol. 11, bulletin 8, January
1945.

27 Snell notes a similar case of a single, elderly man who spent winters
living with a Vancouver friend and summers camping in the interior
of the province until he became ill from gastritis and malnutrition.
The Citizen's Wage, 67.

28 Knight, *Along the No. 20 Line*, 59.

29 These locations are taken from past and current places of residence
listed in applications to Victoria's civic Old Men's Home, VCA-CR.

30 Pat Roy relates the coastal climate to unemployed men. "Vancouver:
'The Mecca of the Unemployed.'"

31 I base my description of this urban male environment on the following
sources: Anderson, "Sharks and Red Herrings," 43–84; Grainger,
Woodsmen of the West, 11–17; Knight, *Along the No. 20 Line*, 55, 59.
McDonald's *Making Vancouver* gives a good portrait of this part of
Vancouver, drawing mostly on Grainger but pulling out the ethnic and
racial elements. Guest links Hastings Street and the life histories of male
residents at Taylor Manor in "Taylor Manor," 39–40.

32 Knight, *Along the No. 20 Line*, 50–5; Wynn, "The Rise of Vancouver,"
89–90; Vancouver Medical Health Officer annual reports cited in
McDonald, *Making Vancouver*, 223.

33 Knight, *Along the No. 20 Line*, 50–5. Although McDonald refers to the cabins used by single working men in *Making Vancouver*, the best description is given to us by Knight.

34 McDonald, *Making Vancouver*, 215–16.

35 Wynn, "The Rise of Vancouver," 135.

36 BCA, GR 289, Box 6, File 2, Government Agent, Smithers to P. Walker, 18 September 1925.

37 Knight, *A Very Ordinary Life*, 160–1.

38 Cole Harris notes that some old miners from Sandon spent their last years in a shack on the base of Idaho Peak where they had worked as miners in their younger days. "Industry and the Good Life," 205.

39 Snell, *The Citizen's Wage*, 64–5.

40 BCA, GR 289, Box 6, File 1, Government Agent, Nelson to Premier John Oliver, 10 June 1925.

41 Ibid., Box 5, File 4, Government Agent, Nanaimo to P. Walker, 1 May 1924.

42 BCA, GR 150, Box 7, File 5, J. Rogers to McMynn, 23 January 1919; J. Rogers to White, 24 November 1919; White to J. Rogers, 8 December 1919; A. to White, 15 December 1919.

43 BCA, GR 131, Box 4, File 3, Social History of J.P., 23 November 1949.

44 Ibid., Social History of M.E., 13 September 1954.

45 Grainger, *Woodsmen of the West*, and Barman, *The West Beyond the West*, 125.

46 McDonald, *Making Vancouver*, 210.

47 Stormi Stewart, in her study of Ontario's turn-of-the-century Wellington House of Industry, notes that employment was pivotal for men wanting to remain outside the institution. "The Elderly Poor," 224.

48 For a history of retirement see Graebner, *A History of Retirement*. Snell sets the historical argument concerning retirement in the Canadian context in *The Citizen's Wage*, 26–35. I do not deal extensively with retirement in my work because it does not appear to have been a significant stage in the lives of the elderly people whom I study.

49 Chudacoff and Hareven, "From the Empty Nest to Family Dissolution," 69–83.

50 Parr's analysis of textile and furniture makers in Ontario shows that male textile workers who did skilled work at the mills in Paris, Ontario in the 1920s typically retained these high status positions until they were in their seventies. Parr suggests that the place for older workers disappeared with mechanization, standardization, and Taylor efficiency methods. *The Gender of Breadwinners*, 77, 168–70.

51 Stewart describes this pattern in Ontario in "The Elderly Poor," 225.

52 BCA, GR 131, Box 4, File 3, Memo, 10 September 1957.

53 The percentage of unskilled labourers in B.C. was 12 per cent in 1891 and 1921, while national average rose from 7 to 9.5 per cent. Seager, "The Resource Economy," 238.
54 Sager and Baskerville, *Unwilling Idlers*, 44.
55 Weiler, "Family Security or Social Security?" 84. Anderson states that the introduction of compulsory compensation for industrial accidents helped push the aged out of employment markets. "The Impact on the Family Relationships," 41.
56 Stewart found seasonal work patterns for elderly men in Ontario. "The Elderly Poor," 225. Morton also notes that older men worked as long as possible, taking lower paying labour as watchmen, janitors, and sweepers as they were pushed out of work they had performed when younger. *Ideal Surroundings*, 91, 97–8. Snell notes that the elderly were given unskilled, low-paid tasks such as janitorial work. *A Citizen's Wage*, 29.
57 BCA, GR 150, Box 7, File 5, W.D. to J.Roger, 11 August 1919.
58 BCA, GR 131, Box 3, Envelope R, A. Noble to P.Walker, 21 July 1924.
59 VCA-CR, Box 29, File 6, Social Service Report on H.B., 28 May 1945.
60 BCA, GR 289, Box 4, File 3, Government Agent, Cranbrook to P. Walker, 21 October 1926.
61 BCA, GR 150, Box 7, File 5, W.D. to J. Roger, 11 August 1919.
62 Cassidy, *Unemployment and Relief in Ontario*, 37.
63 Phillipson states that the concept of "old men's jobs" persisted in Britain until the mid twenties. *Capitalism and the Construction of Old Age*, 23. Anderson places the demise of this form of work in the late nineteenth century. "The Impact on the Family Relationships," 41.
64 BCA, GR 150, Box 7, File 5, J. Roger to Superintendent, Provincial Police, 23 January 1919 and GR 289, Box 1, File 2, Report by Government Sub Agent, Greenwood, 15 July 1927.
65 BCA, GR 289, Box 7, File 2, Government Agent, Vernon to P. Walker, 16 June 1925 and Government Agent, Vernon to P. Walker, 29 May 1925.
66 VCA-CR, Box 19, File 2, F. M. Preston, City Engineer to the Public Works Committee, 29 January 1926.
67 Michael B. Katz, "Origins of the Institutional State," *Marxist Perspectives*, 1 (Winter 1978): 6–22, cited in Stewart, "The Elderly Poor," 218.
68 Gordon, "Familial Support for the Elderly in the Past," 309.
69 Johnston, "Native People, Settlers and Sojourners," 181.
70 Perry, "'Oh I'm Just Sick of the Faces of Men,'" 40.
71 For a discussion of male versus female life cycles and their impact in old age see Weiler, "Family Security or Social Security?" 80–5.
72 BCA, GR 150, Box 12, File 1, claimant to Minister of Mines, 13 March 1923.
73 Gordon, "Familial Support for the Elderly in the Past."

74 RMC, Rose Manor Minute Book, 1917–1926, minutes of meeting, 7 August 1917.

75 BCA, GR 289, Box 1, File 2, J.M. to P. Walker, 7 November 1927.

76 BCA, GR 496, Box 19, File 10, P. Walker to E. Snowden, 20 August 1943.

77 VCA-CR, Box 22, File 2, R. Felton to E. Snowden, 7 February 1933.

78 Bradbury, *Working Families*, 175–9. Nancy Forestell found that boarding house culture was strong in Timmins in the early twentieth century, with the majority of the houses being operated by women. "Bachelors, Boarding-Houses and Blind Pigs," 260. Parr also notes opportunities for women to take in a small number of boarders or run larger boarding houses in the textile town of Paris and the furniture town of Hanover in Ontario in the 1920s and 1930s. *The Gender of Breadwinners*, 81, 190.

79 BCA, GR 289, Box 7, File 7, Report by Provincial Constable, Fernie, 5 October 1926.

80 Ibid., File 1, Report by Government Agent, Nanaimo, 15 October 1926.

81 Cited in Strong-Boag, *The New Day Recalled*, 43.

82 Hinde, "Stout Ladies and Amazons," 33–58.

83 RMC, Rose Manor Minute Book, 1917–1926, minutes of meeting, 6 May 1919.

84 BCA, GR 289, Box 7, File 8, Government Agent, Golden to P. Walker, 23 October 1922, and J.B. to Dr J. MacLean, Provincial Secretary, 5 October 1922.

85 Ibid., Box 2, File 6, Report by Provincial Police Constable, Greenwood, 22 October 1927.

86 The women's Work Room was evidently a municipal welfare endeavour. VCA-CR, Box 22, File 2, R. Felton to E. Snowden, 7 February 1933.

87 BCA, GR 496, Box 19, File 10, P. Walker to E. Snowden, 20 August 1943.

88 Stewart, "The Elderly Poor," 231.

89 BCA, GR 150, Box 9, File 1, Chief Clerk, Provincial Secretary's office to Mrs W., 8 April 1920.

90 Chudacoff and Hareven, "From the Empty Nest to Family Dissolution," 69–83.

91 BCA, GR 289, Box 4, File 3, E.W.C. to J. A. Buckham, n.d.

92 BCA, GR 150, Box 9, File 1, Government Agent, Nelson to P. Walker, 10 November 1921.

93 Snell, *The Citizen's Wage*, 8.

94 BCA, GR 150, Box 8, File 5, letter from J.A. Fraser, Government Agent, Atlin to the Deputy Provincial Secretary, 31 August 1920.

95 The royal commission on old age pensions in Nova Scotia in 1928–30 found that marriage was an important source of support for the elderly. Cited in Snell, *The Citizen's Wage*, 18. Stewart found that few

couples were committed to the Wellington County House of Industry between 1877 and 1907. "The Elderly Poor," 229.

96 Leydier, "Boarding Home Care for the Aged," 31.

97 Hareven, "Life-Course Transitions and Kin Assistance"; Weiler, "Family Security or Social Security?" See also Townsend, *The Family Life of Old People*, for an excellent sociological study. For Canada see Synge, "Work and Family Support Patterns," 135–44, and Snell, *The Citizen's Wage*, ch. 3.

98 BCA, GR 289, Box 5, File 4, Provincial Constable to Government Agent, Cranbrook, 13 June 1921, and Government Agent, Cranbrook to P. Walker, 11 November 1925.

99 BCA, GR 150, Box 9, File 1, Deputy Provincial Secretary to Royal Jubilee Hospital, 26 March 1920.

100 See Bradbury for an excellent description of how women in Montreal used gardens and livestock as part of their family economy. *Working Families*, 163–7. Nova Scotia's 1930 Commission on Old Age Pensions found that informal income from raising chickens and pigs and growing vegetables was a significant source of income for the elderly. Cited in Morton, *Ideal Surroundings*, 55.

101 Wynn, "The Rise of Vancouver," 86.

102 BCA, GR 289, Box 3, File 7, Supervising Nurse, Cowichan Health Centre, to H.W., 29 May 1925.

103 BCA, GR 289, Box 2, File 6, Report by Provincial Constable, Princeton, 23 August 1927.

104 Parr explores the notion of "respectability." *The Gender of Breadwinners*, 187–205.

105 BCA, GR 289, Box 5, File 3, Government Sub Agent, Merritt to P. Walker, 30 September 1926 and Government Agent, Merritt to Deputy Minister of Finance, 4 May 1921.

106 Ibid., Box 2, File 4, Provincial Constable, Keremeos to Government Agent, Penticton, 20 December 1927.

107 Ibid., Box 5, File 4, Report by Provincial Constable, Nanaimo, 14 November 1925.

108 Ibid., Box 1, File 2, Report by Provincial Constable, Vancouver, 26 August 1925.

109 Ibid., Box 6, File 2, Government Agent, Nanaimo to P. Walker, 25 January 1926.

110 Ibid., Box 2, File 6, M.A. to Government Agent, Alberni, 20 February 1923.

111 Chudacoff and Hareven, "From the Empty Nest to Family Dissolution."

112 See, for example, Smith et al., "The Family Structure of the Older Black Population," 544–65; Anderson, "The Impact on the Family Relations," 51–3.

113 BCA, GR 289, Box 3, File 1, G.R. to Superintendent, Provincial Home, 6 June 1927.

114 Ibid., Box 4, File 3, Government Sub Agent, Wilmer to Deputy Provincial Secretary, 31 December 1923.

115 McLaren, "Family Life," 101.

116 BCA, GR 496, Box 19, File 10, Report by F. Hazzard, Regional Supervisor, 7 December 1943.

117 Stewart, "The Elderly Poor," 227–8; Dillon, "Your Place or Mine?," 13; Morton, "Old Women and Their Place," 15; Anderson, "The Impact on the Family Relationships," 51.

118 BCA, GR 289, Box 1, File 7, F. Mutrie, Mothers Pensions Board to P. Walker, 24 September 1927.

119 Anderson, "The Impact on the Family Relationships," 50.

120 BCA, GR 289, Box 7, File 8, Report by Provincial Constable, Nanaimo, 4 October 1926.

121 VCA-CR, Box 24, File 3.

122 BCA, GR 289, Box 1, File 5, Report by Provincial Constable, Fernie, 8 October 1927.

123 Ibid., Box 2, File 4, Report by Provincial Constable, Kamloops, 22 April 1927.

124 Ibid., Box 1, File 10, Report by Provincial Constable, Hazelton District, 7 July 1927.

125 A number of historians have found evidence of greater support for mothers: Stewart, "The Elderly Poor," 22; Katz, *Poverty and Policy*, 122–3; Crowther, *The Workhouse System*, 234.

126 RMC, Minute Book for Home for Aged and Infirm Women beginning April 1901, minutes of meeting, 31 July 1901, and minutes of meeting, 3 September 1901.

127 RMC, Minute Book for Aged and Infirm Women's Home commencing April 1908, minutes of meeting, 2 May 1916.

128 See Townsend, *The Family Life of Old People*, 28–37.

129 BCA, GR 289, Box 2, File 10, F.U. to P. Walker, 19 September 1927.

130 BCA, GR 496, Box 10, File 7, E.B. to H.G. Perry, Minister of Education, 16 March 1945.

131 Anderson, "The Impact on the Family Relationships."

132 Conrad, "Sundays Always Make Me Think of Home," 1–16.

133 BCA, GR 289, Box 3, File 3, Report by Provincial Corporal, Vancouver District, 17 February 1926.

134 Ibid., File 4, Report by Provincial Constable, Port Alice, 17 February 1927.

135 Morton, *Ideal Surroundings*, especially ch. 2.

136 Snell, *The Citizen's Wage*, 60–7.

137 The theoretical literature about community is extensive. For the purposes of this chapter I have found most useful Cohen's *The Symbolic Construction of Community*.

138 BCA, GR 131, Box 3, Envelope B, Government Agent, Vernon to Superintendent, Provincial Home, 29 September 1924.

139 Ibid., Box 4, File 6, Memo by H.S., Social Worker, Social Welfare Branch, 29 September 1924 and M.R. to Department of Social Welfare, Kamloops, 20 January 1961.

140 BCA, GR 289, Box 5, File 3, Report by W.B., 30 September 1926.

141 Ibid., Box 4, File 3, E.C. to J. Buckham, n.d.

142 Ibid., F.C., J.C., and E.M. to Hon A.R. Manson, Attorney General, 4 August 1923.

143 Danysk makes this point for prairie community culture. *Hired Hands*, 64–81, 142–71.

144 BCA, GR 289, Box 3, File 1, M.M. and J.L. to R. Bruhn, 1 March 1927.

145 Danysk notes the responsibility that local people, particularly women, were willing to take for bachelors. "A Bachelor's Paradise," 160–1.

146 Snell, *The Citizen's Wage*, 65–6.

147 BCA, GR 150, Box 7, File 5, J. Rogers to McMynn, 23 January 1919; J. Rogers to White, 24 November 1919; White to J. Rogers, 8 December 1919; A. to White, 15 December 1919.

148 Jeremy Mouat situates this female work within the context of a broad expectation that women would bring domesticity and compassionate care to the western province. *Roaring Days*, 114–15.

149 BCA, GR 131, Box 3, Envelope R, M.M. to F.R., 28 February 1923.

150 BCA, GR 289, Box 1, File 5, Report by Provincial Constable, Quesnel, 1 December 1927.

151 Ibid., Box 7, File 8, Government Agent, Golden to Deputy Provincial Secretary, 17 March 1925.

152 Ibid., Box 3, File 3, Report by Corporal, Provincial Police, Vancouver, 17 February 1926.

153 Wynn, "The Rise of Vancouver," 129–45.

154 Margaret Stacey uses this term in Dennis and Daniels, "Community and the Social Geography of Victorian Cities," 201–24.

155 VCA-CR, Box 33, File 4, Report by Field Service Staff Member, Social Welfare Department, circa 1945–50.

156 Harney, "Men Without Women," 22.

157 BCA, GR 289, Box 4, File 1, G.B. to Deputy Provincial Secretary, 31 January 1925.

158 BCA, GR 150, Box 13, File 3, L.W., Secretary, Ladies' Benevolent Society, Fernie to Government Agent, Fernie, 5 July 1921; Government Agent, Fernie to P. Walker, 11 July 1921.

159 VCA-CR, Box 22, File 2, R. Felton to E. Snowden, 7 February 1933.

160 BCA, GR 1249, Box 2, File 9, Provincial Old Age Pension Department, List of Old Age Pensioners Requesting Medical Attention and Hospitalization, 5 February 1937.

161 McLaren, "Family Life," 101.

162 Morton, *Ideal Surroundings*, 52.

163 Under the terms of the 1871 Municipalities Act local governments in British Columbia were responsible for the destitute residents in their region. But throughout most of the period covered by this chapter the City of Vancouver was the only municipality with an organized relief department. Moreover, much of the province was unorganized territory and hence health and social welfare was the responsibility of the provincial government in these areas. The clearest articulation of the way in which the fund operated can be found in the following document: BCA, GR 150, Box 14, File 12, P. Walker to Captain C.S. Leary, 19 January 1927.

164 This interpretation of paternalism is based on Finlayson's discussion of the subject. *Citizen, State and Social Welfare in Britain*, 19–106.

165 BCA, GR 289, Box 6, File 5, M.L.A. to Provincial Secretary, 8 December 1925; Box 3, File 7, Report by Provincial Constable, Yahk, 29 December 1926.

166 Ibid., Box 3, File 4, Government Agent, Cranbrook to P. Walker, 23 August 1927.

167 Roberts, *Paternalism in Early Victorian England*, 180–1, 270.

168 BCA, GR 289, Box 5, File 3, Government Sub Agent, Merritt to P. Walker, 30 September 1926.

169 Ibid., Box 6, File 2, Government Agent, Smithers to P. Walker, 18 September 1925.

170 BCA, GR 150, Box 7, File 6, Chief Clerk, Provincial Secretary's office to Chief Constable, Nanaimo, 9 July 1919.

171 BCA, GR 150, Box 14, File 12, P. Walker to Captain C.S. Leary, 19 January 1927.

172 Ibid., Box 5, File 2, P. Walker to Superintendent, Provincial Police, 16 October 1924.

173 BCA, GR 289, Box 3, File 7, Supervising Nurse, Cowichan Health Centre to H.W., 29 May 1925, with reference to a letter from Provincial Constable, Duncan Station to Division "A," District Victoria, dated 19 September 1924.

174 BCA, GR 150, Box 11, File 4, Government Agent, Smithers to P. Walker, 23 August 1922.

175 BCA, GR 289, Box 1, File 7, Report by Provincial Constable, Nakusp, 26 October 1925.

176 Documents found in the Saanich Municipal Archives show that the association was active from March 1931 (and likely earlier) until at

least 1940. SMA, Clerk's Department, Box 43, File 4 and Box 62A, File 5.

177 Cassidy, *Public Health and Welfare Reorganization*, 44–5. From 1911 the secretary of the Friendly Help Association was also Victoria's city relief officer. In Saanich, the welfare association received financial and practical municipal support from the municipality, local businesses, and women's groups.

178 Finlayson, *Citizen, State and Social Welfare*, 199.

179 Taylor, "The Urban West, Public Welfare."

180 "Home for Old and Destitute Becomes Crying Need," *Daily Province*, 4 September 1909.

181 Guest, "Taylor Manor," 17.

182 Knight, *A Very Ordinary Life*, 225.

183 McDonald, *Making Vancouver*, 221.

184 BCA, GR 289, Box 1, File 5, District Secretary to M.E. Smith, 2 February 1927.

185 VCA-CR, Box 22, File 21, R.D. Felton to Ald. Alex Peden, 7 December 1932.

186 Bryden gives a detailed description of the political process that accompanied the introduction of old age pensions and pension administration. *Old Age Pensions*, 63–74, 100–1.

187 This interpretation of corporatism is based on the ideas of Harold Perkin. See Perkin, *The Rise of Professional Society*, ch. 8.

188 Bryden gives an analysis of the calculations that underpinned old age pension payments and of the relative monetary value of the pension at different times. *Old Age Pensions*, 62, 92–3. Struthers graphically describes the hardships Ontario's pensioners faced in the 1940s. *The Limits of Affluence*, 73–4.

189 This policy shift is detailed in Mathewson, "Old Age Pensions in British Columbia," 44–5.

190 Amy Edwards is an example of B.C.'s new breed of welfare professionals and was one of the first geriatric "experts" in the province. She moved to the Pensions Department in 1943. Cassidy, "Personnel Changes in British Columbia," and Mathewson, "Old Age Pensions in British Columbia," 44–5.

191 This is a recurring theme in professional writing about the aged. For example, "Annual Report of the Old-age Pension Board," SP, vol. 2, 1945, T-12.

192 "Report of the Social Assistance Branch, 1944–45," SP, vol. 2, 1946, R-45.

193 Snell, *The Citizen's Wage*, 188.

194 Pensions had a huge impact on the quality of life for Britain's elderly. There, old age pensions were introduced in 1908. Four years later Poor

Law outrelief payments had dropped by 95 per cent. Anderson, "The Impact on the Family Relationships," 43–4.

195 James Snell notes that B.C. pension administrators were particularly sympathetic toward their elderly clients. *The Citizen's Wage*, 188. This was not the case elsewhere in Canada, where old age pension administration was harsh and judgmental in its dealings with aged applicants. See Snell, *The Citizen's Wage*, 188–92 and Struthers, *The Limits of Affluence*, 63–9 for descriptions of Ontario's punitive pensions policy.

196 BCA, GR 289, Box 1, File 2, Report by Government Sub Agent, Greenwood, 15 July 1927, and Government Agent, Penticton to P. Walker, 20 July 1927.

197 Old-Age Pension Board Report in "Annual Report of the Social Welfare Branch of the Department of Health and Welfare, 1950," SP, vol. 2, 1951, R-59. James Snell found that pensions politicized the elderly, creating a new concept of the rights of "senior citizens." *The Citizen's Wage*, 10–11.

198 For example, Townsend, "The Structured Dependency of the Elderly," 16–19.

199 Anderson, "The Impact on the Family Relationships," 44; Crowther, *The Workhouse System*, 219.

200 Bryden argues that pensions made it possible for some elderly to avoid or postpone entering an institution. *Old Age Pensions*, 35. Strong-Boag makes the same point in reference to an institution in Winnipeg. *The New Day Recalled*, 189.

201 Struthers, "Regulating the Elderly," 235–55.

202 Snell sets these developments in the national context. *The Citizen's Wage*, 9–10.

203 For examples of this argument see Phillipson, *Capitalism and the Construction of Old Age,* and Townsend, "The Structured Dependency of the Elderly," 6–28.

204 BCA, GR 131, Box 4, File 3, Social History of J.P., 23 November 1949.

205 BCA, GR 150, Box 7, File 5, J. Rogers to McMynn, 23 January 1919; J. Rogers to White, 24 November 1919; White to J. Rogers, 8 December 1919; A. to White, 15 December 1919.

CHAPTER TWO

1 Markus uses this notion in a slightly different fashion, to speak about space and power in terms of institutional space. I am borrowing his concept and applying it more broadly to the social and cultural place of the old age home in the larger community. Markus, *Buildings and Power*, 5.

2 Christie, *They Do It With Mirrors*, 84.

3 There is a vast literature on this subject. Among the books that I found useful were King, *Buildings and Society,* and Markus, *Buildings and Power.*

4 For an extensive body of material on this subject see *Royal Architectural Institute of Canada Journal,* ser. 444, vol. 39, no. 8 (August 1962). In addition to an article on Victoria's Matson Lodge, there are general discussions concerning the architecture of old age homes, and specific articles on the Saskatchewan Geriatric Centre, Toronto's Salvation Army Arthur Meighen Lodge, Oshawa's Hillsdale Manor Home for the Aged, and the Nipponia Home for the Aged in Beamsville, Ontario.

5 Cook, "'A Quiet Place ... To Die,'" 25. In the latter decades of the nineteenth century benevolent homes for the aged were established across the United States and in central Canada. In Minnesota, for example, nine such homes had been established by 1900. Nash and McClure, "Aging in Retrospect," 2.

6 Cassidy, *Public Health and Welfare Reorganization,* 38–40.

7 Forbes et al., *Institutionalization of the Elderly in Canada,* 11. For Sweden see Sundstrom, "Family and State," 169–96. In Britain, the replacement of older poorhouses by new residential homes was slowed by a lack of funds, but a total of 1,184 homes for the old and the handicapped opened in England and Wales between 1948 and 1960. Figures cited in Means and Smith, *The Development of Welfare Services,* 177. For background to the links between the growth of private residential accommodation for aged Americans under the 1935 Social Security Act or Medicare and Medicaid in the 1960s see Achenbaum, *Shades of Grey,* 40, and Achenbaum, *Old Age in the New Land,* 151.

8 Davies, "Old Age in British Columbia."

9 VCA, *City Reports,* "Report of the Committee on Old Men's Home," 6 January 1892, 63–5.

10 VCA-CR, Box 3, File 3, "Home Committees' Report," 12 June 1893; Box 9, File 1, "Report of the Cemetery Committee," 18 April 1904. The building was located in Block "R" of the cemetery, among "some of the choicest lots in the cemetery," and is marked on a fire insurance map of the Ross Bay Cemetery dated August 1904, VCA.

11 VCA, *City Reports,* "Report of the Home for Aged and Infirm, for year ending Dec 31, 1984."

12 VCA-CR, Box 9, File 1, 1 April and 17 April 1906, "Reports of the Home Committee." Also, OB-DHM, 1.

13 "New Home Ready for the Old Men," *Victoria Daily Colonist,* 30 May 1906, 10.

14 VCA, *City Reports,* "Report of the Home Manager," 17 March 1920.

15 Haber, *Beyond Sixty-Five*, 106. Ottawa's Protestant Home for the Aged was moved outside city limits in 1889. Cook, ""A Quiet Place ... to Die,'" 28.

16 "A Plea for the Aged Men," *Daily Province*, 20 May 1905, 13.

17 The terms "derived" and "designed" come from Thompson and Goldin, *The Hospital*, xxvii. Rothman found that the eighteenth-century American almshouse was modelled on a family dwelling. *The Discovery of the Asylum*, 42–3.

18 This description is based on a photograph of the Old Men's Home found in the Havard Memoirs, OB-DHM, and "New Home Ready for the Old Men," *Victoria Daily Colonist*, 30 May 1906, 10.

19 VCA, Fire insurance map, Old Men's Home, 1938, and OB-DHM, 2–3, and VCA-CR, Box 18, File 3.

20 The infirmary was built with funds raised by subdividing property at the Home. VCA, Minutes of the Meeting of the Social Welfare and Aged Men's Home Committee, 20 July 1951.

21 Cassidy, *Public Health and Welfare Reorganization*, 45.

22 The description of the Kamloops Home interior is based on Isobel Harvey's 1945 detailed study of provincial institutions for chronic patients. BCLL, Harvey, "Study of Chronic Diseases."

23 Markus, *Buildings and Power*, 129.

24 BCA, GR 131, Box 2, File 12, Annual Report, Provincial Home, 1 April 1950 to 31 March 1951.

25 BCA, GR 496, Box 54, File 1, Noble to Walker, 16 July 1941.

26 BCA, photo number 66438, and BCA, GR 496, Box 54, File 1, Noble to Walker, 16 July 1941.

27 BCA, GR 277, Box 3, File 3, plan and description of the Provincial Home from the 1950s.

28 "A Plea for the Aged Men, "*Daily Province*, 20 May 1905, 13; "May Turn Ranch into Home for Aged," *Daily Province*, 21 August 1906, 1.

29 Information about Vancouver's Old People's Home is extremely limited. Two master's theses done by UBC students in the 1940s provide valuable information about the history of the Home. Mathewson, "Old Age Pensions in British Columbia," 4, puts the building's date at 1913; Guest says the Home was constructed in 1915. "Taylor Manor," 12.

30 Knight, *Along the No. 20 Line*.

31 "Home for old and destitutes becoming crying need in Vancouver Problem of Housing our Dependents," *Daily Province*, 4 September 1909.

32 "New Old People's Home," *Daily Province*, 23 June 1915, 1.

33 The Home had space for three married couples but the annual reports do not indicate whether any married couples were resident. Mathewson, "Old Age Pensions in British Columbia," 4; Guest, "Taylor Manor," 15.

34 Mathewson, "Old Age Pensions in British Columbia," 4; Guest, "Taylor Manor," 20.

35 The provincial government originally planned to re-establish the facility in a more modern building, but this did not take place. BCA, GR 277, Box 5, File 2, Law, "Report on the Provincial Infirmaries, 1954," 1; McFarland, "The Care of the Chronically Ill," 23. For a history of the evolution of the workhouse infirmary into public hospitals in England and Wales see Crowther, *The Workhouse System*, 156–90.

36 My description of Marpole Infirmary is based on the following sources: BCA, GR 496, Box 23, File 12, "Report of the Provincial Infirmary, Marpole, for the year ending March 31, 1941"; BCLL, Harvey, "Study of Chronic Diseases," 8–9; BCA, GR 277, Box 5, File 1, D. Turnbull, 21 July 1950, "Memorandum of Visit to Infirmaries on July 19, 1950," Box 3, File 4, L.F. Detwiller, "Report on Survey of Provincial Infirmary, Marpole," August 1955; "No Tears, No Regrets as Old Infirmary Shuts," *Vancouver Sun*, 7 May 1965.

37 Very little is known about the Provincial Home for Incurables or its inhabitants until after 1935, and thus my discussion about the facility concentrates on a period of expansion and change. McFarland notes that standards of care and treatment at the institution were very low before 1937. "The Care of the Chronically Ill," 60. Patient and staff numbers are based on BCA, GR 496, Box 47, File 8, H.M. Cassidy, "Report on the Home for Incurables," 25 January 1938, 1; BCA, GR 496, Box 47, File 9, Zella M. Collins, "Report Prepared for Advisory Board, Provincial Infirmary," 6 March 1939.

38 Province of British Columbia, *Public Health Nursing*.

39 SMA, Vertical Subject Files, Hospitals, "A Brief Summary of the History of the Saanich War Memorial Health Centre"; BCA, GR 281, Register of Licenses for Private Hospitals, 151, 166; SMA, Clerk's Department, Box 87, File 3, Clerk of the Municipal Council to W. Greene, 8 August 1946, and Box 132, File 2, Reeve, Corporation of the District of Saanich to Nixon, 30 October 1952.

40 In 1917 the VGH took over the bankrupt Grand Hotel and built a Military Annex. These details come from McFarland, "The Care of the Chronically Ill," 23, 49, and VANCA, Series 452, Box 106 F2, File 6, M. McKenna, "Short History of the Hospital Annex, Vancouver General Hospital," 1963.

41 VCA-CR, Box 18, File 3, G. McGregor to R.H.B Kerr, 10 April 1924; "Health Committee Report," 9 June 1924; Box 18, File 5, "Health Committee Report," 9 February 1925; Box 24, File 4, D. Muire to J.A. Worthington, 18 February 1938.

42 Gresko, "Salomée Valois."

43 VCA-CR, Box 18, File 3, G. McGregor to R.H.B. Kerr, 10 April 1924.

44 This interpretation was suggested to me by Sheila Norton.

45 BCA, GR 496, Box 49, File 8, P. Ward, Memo, 2 June 1942.

46 VCA-CR, Box 18, File 3, G. McGregor to R.H.B. Kerr, 10 April 1924. BCA, GR 496, Box 49, File 8, P. Ward, Memo, 2 June 1942, quotes from the "Report of the Vancouver General Hospital *Survey* Commission upon the Hospital Situation of Greater Vancouver, 1930."

47 VCA, *City Reports*, "Health Officer's Report, 1922." From 1925 all city cases went to Mrs Ross at the Maple Rest Home.

48 SMA, Clerk's Department, Box 62, File 1, G.E. Chapman to W. Greene, 23 April 1940.

49 McFarland, "The Care of the Chronically Ill," 23. McFarland reports that a small number of patients were also placed in the Royal Derby and Florence Nightingale private hospitals in the first years.

50 VCA, *City Reports*, "Health Officer's Reports," 1920, 1924.

51 Other historians have observed these contours of philanthropic work for aged and respectable women. See Cook, "'A Quiet Place ... to Die'," 25–40; Cole, *The Journey of Life*, 173; Haber, *Beyond Sixty-Five*, 92–3. Ida Gould, in her 1928 history of the Home, makes it clear in her descriptions of the first residents that this was a charitable enterprise designed to care for respectable women who, through no fault of their own, had fallen on hard times. *History of the Aged and Infirm Women's Home*, 3–9.

52 Gould, *History of the Aged and Infirm Women's Home*, 9; BCA, photo C-08979

53 Gould, *History of the Aged and Infirm Women's Home*, 12–14.

54 RMC, Minute Book of the Aged Women's Home started May 1944, newsclipping from local newspaper, editorial, 10 April 1948.

55 Women at the Home always had their own chairs; in 1938 the dining room tables were cut to seat six. Details about the Home from RMC, Minute Book of the Aged Women's Home started 5 May 1936, minutes of meeting, 7 July 1936; minutes of meeting, 17 February 1938; minutes of meeting, 5 December 1939.

56 RMC, Minute Book of the Aged Women's Home started 5 May 1936, minutes of meeting, 1 December 1936, 2 February 1937, and 6 February 1937; Minute Book of the Aged Women's Home started May 1944, minutes of meeting, 1 November 1949.

57 RMC, Minute Book of the Aged Women's Home started 5 May 1936, minutes of meeting, 6 September 1937.

58 VCA, *City Reports*, "Health Officer's Reports," 1923, 1928.

59 For examples of this, RMC, Minute book for Aged and Infirm Women's Home commencing April 1908, minutes of meeting, 2 February 1915.

60 VCA-CR, Box 19, File 5, A. Whittier to Dr A. Price, 17 December 1926.

61 Religious groups represented by the women included the Daughters of Rebecca, the Methodist, Baptist, Presbyterian, Roman Catholic, and Reformed Episcopalian denominations, and Jews. At the homes in Ottawa studied by Sharon Cook men took the administrative positions and played a central role in running the two charitable homes for the elderly in the city. "'A Quiet Place ... to Die,'" 25–40.

62 RMC, Minute Book for Home for Aged and Infirm Women beginning April 1901, minutes of meeting, 5 October 1901.

63 There is little biographical information available about these women. Harriet Carne is the subject of a chapter titled "The Oldest Lady in Victoria" in Lugrin, *The Pioneer Women of Vancouver Island*, 252–8. Helen Grant, first president of the Home, was also Victoria's second female school trustee. Other women who were prominent in the early history of the Home included Mrs I.A. Gould, Mrs Charles Hayward, Mrs Lawrence Goodacre, Mrs W.L. Clay, and Mrs Amelia Whittier. There were two women with the surname Clay involved over the years, and two Grants, Mrs W. Grant, in 1938 the only surviving member of the original committee, and Mrs H. Grant, who joined in 1917. RMC, Whittier, "History of Aged and Infirm Women's Home."

64 RMC, Rose Manor Minute Book, 1917–1926, minutes of meeting, 3 May 1921.

65 In 1884 only 106 of the 1,767 Chinese residents in Victoria were women. Cited in Lai, "From Self-segregation to Integration," 53. While I did not find regulations prohibiting men of specific ethnic backgrounds from entering Victoria's Old Men's Home, the absence of Chinese men from the facility is striking, considering the destitute circumstances of single indigent men in the Chinese community. My conclusion is that Chinese men were probably not permitted to enter the Old Men's Home. The Provincial Home Act of 1893 excluded Chinese from admission to Kamloops facility. Li, *The Chinese in Canada*, 37–9.

66 Lai, "From Self-segregation to Integration," 54.

67 Ibid., 56–61.

68 Ibid., 61–2.

69 Province of British Columbia, *Hospital Statistics*, 1942, 23.

70 BCA, GR 2577, Box 10, Files 9 and 10, Chinese Community Hospital, Correspondence, 1962–1963.

71 BCA, GR 1582, Box 182, File 376.

72 McFarland, "The Care of the Chronically Ill," 15, 51.

73 Private maternity hospitals in Vancouver virtually disappeared between 1919 and 1939. Strong-Boag and McPherson, "The Confinement of Women," 142–74.

74 For example, three women, the Misses J. and A. M. Archibald and Miss C. M. Grimmer, opened the Victoria Private Hospital in 1913. In

1921 the hospital was taken over by Miss D.L. Exley, who continued
to operate the facility after her 1923 marriage. In 1925 the Victoria Private Hospital moved from its Rockland Avenue location to Yates Street.
It closed two years later. BCA, GR 281, 3.

75 Province of British Columbia, *Hospital Service and Costs*, 1934, 11.
76 McFarland, "The Care of the Chronically Ill," 41–3.
77 Ibid.
78 VANCA, J.S. Matthews files, n.d.
79 VCA-CR, Box 22, File 4, Aldermen McGavin and McGodd, "Minority
   Report concerning Maple Rest Nursing Home," 21 August 1933;
   Minutes of a Meeting of the Health (Special) Committee, 31 July 1933.
80 A significant exception to this trend was in the field of mental health.
   In 1945 there was only a small unit for elderly patients at Essondale,
   the provincial mental health facility in Port Coquitlam. A branch was
   established in 1948 in a former military hospital in Vernon and another
   three years later in Terrace. By 1958 these facilities had 1,100 elderly
   patients, in contrast to 260 beds in the provincial infirmary system.
   Elmore, "Discharge Planning in Homes for the Aged," 14–18; "Annual
   Report of the Social Welfare Branch for the Department of Health and
   Welfare, 1949," SP, vol. 2, 1950, R-51.
81 The Sisters had approached the provincial government for financial
   assistance in opening a chronic care facility to help ease the need for
   beds for hospital clearance cases. BCA, GR 496, Box 47, File 9,
   Minutes of the Advisory Board Meeting, Provincial Infirmary, 17 July
   1941; SSAA, Mount Saint Mary's Correspondence, Sisters of Saint Ann
   to G.M. Weir, 4 April 1938; G.M. Weir to Rev. Sister Mary Elfreda,
   13 May 1941.
82 Sleek and sparsely decorated, the tuberculosis wing was also a visual
   embodiment of the principles of modern science. Thompson and
   Goldin, *The Hospital*, 190, 207; Forty, "The Modern Hospital in
   England and France," 61–93.
83 Haney is in the Fraser Valley outside Vancouver. It opened in 1935
   as a hospital camp for men on relief. Patient release figures are
   quite high, which suggests that it did not serve as a custodial institution. However, it appears that the majority of the thirteen men that
   died at Allco and Camp 202 at Deroche in 1935 were elderly,
   indicating that some elderly infirm men on relief found shelter in
   these institutions before Allco became a branch of the Provincial Infirmary. BCA, GR 496, Box 15, File 8, J. A. West to Dr J.G. McCammon,
   30 January 1936.
84 There are a number of hints that many of the men at Allco were alco-
   holics, which may account for the willingness of government administrators to place them in this facility. BCA, GR 678, Box 5, File 15,

"Report on Visits to the Marpole and Allco Infirmaries, February 13th and 14th, 1958."

85 My description of Allco is based on the following sources: BCLL, Harvey, "A Study of Chronic Diseases"; McFarland, "The Care of the Chronically Ill"; "Allco and Marpole," *Vancouver Province*, 29 January 1947, 4; BCA, GR 277, Box 5, File 1, D. Turnbull, "Memorandum of Visit to Infirmaries on July 19, 1950," 21 July 1950.

86 VCA-CR, Box 28, File 4, "Report of the Post-War Rehabilitation Committee," 6 November 1943, and File 6, "Report of the Social Welfare Committee," 1 March 1944; SMA, Clerk's Department, Box 78, File 3, M. Hunter to W. Greene, 26 January 1944; BCA, Local Council of Women, Victoria, Add. MSS. 2818, Box 1, File 27, "Report by the Committee to the Mayor and Aldermen, City of Victoria."

87 Gorge Road Hospital Files, Gayton, "Gorge Road Hospital History," 2.

88 As described in n80, provincial mental health facilities were established in former military hospitals in Vernon and Terrace.

89 Doreen Heelas, "Haven in the Valley," *Daily Province*, 27 January 1951, 8.

90 SMA, Clerk's Department, Box 91, File 1, from C.P. Ennals to E. G. Snowden, 11 March 1946; Reeve, Corporation of the District of Saanich to G.H.S. Dinsmore, 25 April 1946. Three years later the municipality made an unsuccessful attempt to interest the Salvation Army in setting up a home for the aged in the hospital building at the Gordon Head Army Camp, the present site of the University of Victoria. SMA, Clerk's Department, Box 110, File 6, Reeve, Corporation of the District of Saanich to C.J. Miller, 24 October 1949, and Miller to the Municipal Clerk, 1 December 1944.

91 In 1950, for example, Saanich's municipal council stated that they did not believe that nursing homes were a municipal responsibility. SMA, Clerk's Department, Box 118, File 3, Reeve, Corporation of the District of Saanich to G. Harris, 22 March 1950.

92 Gorge Road Hospital Files, Gayton, "Gorge Road Hospital History," 2.

93 "Annual Report of the Social Welfare Branch," 1950, SP, vol. 2, 1951, R-65.

94 McFarland, "The Care of the Chronically Ill," 55.

95 Berton, "25 Pensioners Happy at Mother Fowler's," 13.

96 Details on this institutional expansion come from: BCA, GR 496, Box 49, File 5, "Report on Statistics and Administration of the Welfare Institutions Licensing Act for the year ended 31st December, 1944"; GR 2720, Box 1, Report, 15 April 1948; Province of British Columbia, *Hospital Statistics*, 1943, 25; SMA, Clerk's Department, Box 132, File 1, "Report of the Salvation Army Social Services Activities for the Year Ended December 31, 1951," 2.

97 The Anglican Church, Diocese of British Columbia, was also involved in the Twilight Homes Project, which opened a "Welcome Room" for women pensioners in downtown Victoria in 1948, and in the Dawson Heights Cottages in 1949. The architectural notes on the Home are taken from a promotional brochure produced by Home administrators in the 1990s.

98 Diocese of British Columbia Archives, Box 1, File 1, Text 343, Minutes of the Board of Governors of the Caroline Macklem Home, 1950–1953.

99 Townsend, *The Last Refuge*, 109–12.

100 SSAA, Series 61, Box 1, Chair, Mount St Francis Advisory Committee to R.W. Diamond, 30 January 1950.

101 SSAA, Series 61, Box 1, Sister Mary Mildred, Provincial Superior, "Survey of Project for Rest Home for Aged Pensioners, Nelson, B.C.," 2 December 1946.

102 "The Salvation Army Matson Lodge," *Royal Architectural Institute of Canada Journal*, ser. 444, vol. 39, no. 8 (August 1962), 35–7.

103 "Dream Home for Old Folks," *Daily Province*, 26 February 1944.

104 "Where old people are understood," 29. I surmise that the "recently opened boarding home" described by Bernice Leydier must be the Icelandic Home. Leydier, "Boarding Home Care for the Aged," 62–4.

105 For a parallel process in another industry see Cohen, "The Decline of Women in Canadian Dairying," 307–34.

106 Statistics taken from BCA, GR 281, Register of Private Hospitals, and Province of British Columbia, *Hospital Statistics*, 1935–1939.

107 SMA, Clerk's Department, Box 132, File 2, Reeve, Corporation of the District of Saanich to Nixon, 30 October 1952; Box 1, File 5, Planning Commission (subject files), Application for rezoning, 13 November 1957. Province of British Columbia, *Hospital Statistics*, 1958, 45.

108 These details are taken from BCA, GR 678, Box 1, File 6, memorandum by James Mainguy, 19 July 1956.

109 SMA, Clerk's Department, Box 95, File 6, E. Page to J.B. Tribe, 6 December 1947.

110 BCA, GR 2720, Box 1, File titled "Boarding Homes and Nursing Homes," Report, 15 April 1948; SMA, Clerk's Department, Box 62, File 1, J.B. Tribe to E. Pringle, 20 November 1940.

111 BCA, GR 496, Box 49, File 5, "Report on Statistics and Administration of the Welfare Institutions Licensing Act for the year ended 31st December, 1944."

112 McFarland, "The Care of the Chronically Ill," 75.

113 Leydier, "Boarding Home Care for the Aged," 47, 61, 67.

114 SMA, Clerk's Department, Box 95, File 6, J.L. Gayton to Reeve and Council, Corporation of Saanich, 4 July 1947.

115 BCA, GR 496, Box 49, File 8, B. Snider to E. Pringle, 26 January 1939.

116 McFarland, "The Care of the Chronically Ill," 75.

117 The description of the home for retired women, which was likely one of those surveyed by Leydier, is taken from "Soroptimist House Friendly Haven for Retired Women," *Vancouver News Herald*, 2 April 1947, 7. The rest of the details come from Leydier, "Boarding Home Care for the Aged," 61–9. Leydier makes the point that the use of borrowed buildings was a direct consequence of post-war housing and economics: the demand for all levels of residential accommodation for the elderly in B.C. was increasing, but the high cost of construction materials inhibited building.

118 McFarland notes the historical pattern of leasing beds in private hospitals for the chronically ill. "The Care of the Chronically Ill," 23.

CHAPTER THREE

1 For the United States see Haber, *Beyond Sixty-Five*, ch. 5. For Australia see Parker, *The Elderly and Residential Care*, ch. 2. For Britain, the best source is Means and Smith, *From Poor Law to Community Care*.

2 For example, Wagner, "New Patterns for Old Age," 63–71.

3 Farquhar, "Services for the Aged," 109–12.

4 Creighton, "Birthdays Don't Count," 37–40, and Letter to the Editor, *The Canadian Doctor*, 4.

5 BCLL, Harvey, "Study of Chronic Diseases," 28.

6 "In a Shameful Condition," *Province*, 21 January 1947, 4; "That Place at Marpole," *Vancouver News Herald*, 23 January 1947, 4; "Our Shameful Neglect," *Vancouver Sun*, 30 January 1947, 4; "Allco and Marpole," *Province*, 29 January 1947, 4; "Chronic Misery," *Vancouver Sun*, 6 February 1947, 4. Change in Britain was apparently precipitated by a series of letters published in the *Manchester Guardian* in 1943 that condemned public assistance institutions, the direct descendent of the poorhouse. Samson, *Old Age in the New World*, 40–7.

7 For an extended discussion of professionalism see Perkin, *The Rise of Professional Society*.

8 For an excellent analysis of American developments see Achenbaum, *Crossing Frontiers*, and for a very useful introduction to British geriatric specialization, with particular attention to the unique characteristics of Scottish developments and to the role of the National Health Service, see Thane, *Old Age in English History*, ch. 22.

9 The observation about publications is based on my own survey of Canadian medical and social work journals from 1900 to 1950. There were virtually no articles on old age in Canadian medical and social work journals until the final Depression years. Canadian politicians and

others looking at the elderly focused on poverty and pension reform. Guest, *The Emergence of Social Security*, 74–9.

10 In 1953 the federal government set up the Joint Committee on Old Age Security of the Senate and House of Commons, the first national committee to study aging. Novak, *Aging and Society*, 15–17, outlines early developments. See Rudy, *For Such a Time as Time*, 142–7, for the history of geriatric studies in Ontario.

11 "Annual Report of the Social Welfare Branch of the Department of Health and Welfare, 1950," SP, vol. 2, 1951, R-63–64. For a reference to training for work with the aged in Britain see Means and Smith, *From Poor Law to Community Care*, 195–6. Rehabilitative medicine, a medical speciality that expanded during the Second World War, emphasized a broad approach to healing and well-being. Psychiatry, physiotherapy, occupational and speech therapy, social service, guidance and testing, vocational and employment training, recreation, financial assistance, selective placement, and "careful follow-up" were all included under the rubric of rehabilitative medicine. MacQuarrie, "The Care of An Ageing and Disabled Group," 3.

12 I draw on the ideas of Paul Starr here. *The Social Transformation*, 13–21.

13 Dr Harry Cassidy submitted a report on the Home for Incurables to Weir, the provincial secretary, in October 1937. Based in part on observations of Amyot and Ward, this document advocated sweeping changes to the facility. The complete text of this report appears to have been lost. BCA, GR 496, Box 47, File 8, H. Cassidy, "Report on the Home for Incurables," 25 January 1938.

14 BCA, GR 496, Box 23, File 12, C.M. Motherwell, "Annual Report of the Provincial Infirmary for the year 1938–39"; Box 47, File 8, H. Cassidy, "Report on the Home for Incurables," 25 January 1938.

15 BCA, GR 496, Box 23, File 12, C.M. Motherwell, "Annual Report of the Provincial Infirmary for the year 1938–39."

16 I draw here on the ideas of Andrew Abbott concerning the cultural malleability of professional work. *The System of Professionals*, especially ch. 2.

17 BCA, GR 496, Box 23, File 12, C.M. Motherwell, "Annual Report of the Provincial Infirmary for the year 1938–39"; File 12, M. Law, "Annual Report of the Provincial Infirmary for the year ending March 31, 1943"; GR 277, Box 5, File 1, M. Law, "Annual Report on Provincial Infirmaries, 1950."

18 "Annual Report of the Welfare Institutions Licensing Board, 1949," SP, vol. 2, 1951, R 105.

19 Holland, "Our Senior Citizens."

20 BCA, GR 496, Box 47, File 8, H. Cassidy, "Report on the Home for Incurables," 25 January 1938; BCA, GR 496, Box 47, File 9, Zella

M. Collins, "Report Prepared for Advisery Board, Provincial Infirmary." 6 March 1939.

21 BCA, GR 496, Box 48, File 2, P. Ward to P. Walker, 25 May 1943.

22 BCA, GR 678, Box 1, File 6, memo by James Mainguy details the
administrative criteria of these different levels of care, 19 July 1956.

23 BCA, GR 678, Box 1, File 14, F. Heaton to D. Cox, January 1957.

24 BCA, GR 678, Box 43, File 20, Doris E. Mackay, "Survey of the Population of Private Hospitals in B.C.," completed in 1965.

25 BCA, GR 496, Box 23, File 12, "Annual Report of the Provincial Infirmary for the Year, 1938–39"; Box 5, File 5, Office of the Inspector of
Hospitals to P. Walker, 30 May 1944. In 1948 McFarland noted the
Marpole was the only institution in the province that could be classi-
fied as a chronic care hospital. *The Care of the Chronically Ill*, 15.

26 Thane, "Geriatrics."

27 BCA, GR 496, Box 23, File 12, "Report of the Provincial Infirmary for
the year ending March 31, 1946."

28 Ibid., "Annual Report of the Provincial Infirmary for the year ending
March 31, 1942."

29 Ibid., Box 12, File 2, M. Baldwin, "Report on Food Served and
Feeding Facilities, Provincial Home, Kamloops," April 1945.

30 Women, who had a strong position within the field of social work,
benefited from the fact that the new Pattullo government of 1933 was
anxious to base their welfare programs on social work principles and
that there was a shortage of trained social workers during the Depression years. The extreme reluctance of the B.C. government to bring
in trained personnel from outside the province may also have worked
to the advantage of women.

31 Looking at the British situation, Means and Smith tell us that "[r]esi-
dential work with elderly people was seen as 'women's work' in which
the appropriate qualities of warmth, gentleness and good housekeeping
would flow naturally from the right type of applicant with the minimum of instruction." *From Poor Law to Community Care*, 195.

32 Rowe et al., "The Care of the Chronically Ill." Also Barker, "On the
Care of the Aged." Government officials also favoured these qualities in
those who worked with the elderly. For example, "Report of the Social
Assistance Branch, 1944–45," in SP, vol. 2, 1946, R-44. Harvey's report
also stressed the importance of a "pleasant personality" and "understanding and kindness" in caregivers, assuming this person would be
female. BCLL, Harvey, "Study of Chronic Diseases," 9, 22.

33 Reporting a serious lack of communication between field staff, doctors,
and infirmary administrators, Harvey argues that a medical social
worker (always referred to as "she") would be able to act as an inter-
preter between the various parties involved. BCLL, Harvey, "Study of

Chronic Diseases," 12. A 1952 report also saw the social worker as intermediary. BCA, GR 277, Box 7, File 4, A. Mann, "Report concerning a social worker for the Provincial Infirmary," 25 November 1952.

34 BCA, GR 496, Box 23, File 12, "Annual Report of the Provincial Infirmary for the year ending March 31, 1942."

35 May, *Homeward Bound*, 172.

36 Snell discusses the development of the "senior citizen" – both the term and the concept – in Canada. *The Citizen's Wage*, introduction.

37 Names are a useful way of placing institutions within the broader social and cultural milieu that has produced them. Townsend notes similar types of names for post-war old age homes in England and Wales as I found in B.C., but does not speculate as to their meaning. *The Last Refuge*, 112.

38 BCA, GR 678, Box 10, File 26, Donald Cox, "Increasing Attention to Chronic Diseases and Geriatrics," paper presented at the American College of Surgeons Sectional Meeting in Minneapolis, 1948.

39 Rudy, *For Such a Time as This*, appendix A lists all old age homes in Ontario founded between 1837 and 1961.

40 Guest, "Taylor Manor," 25.

41 *Victoria and Vancouver Island Directory (1952)*, 256.

42 Townsend, *The Last Refuge*, 112.

43 Strong-Boag, "Home Dreams."

44 Guest, *The Emergence of Social Security*, 25.

45 BCA, Add. MSS. 2818, File 27, Local Council of Women, Victoria, Temporary Committee to the Mayor of Victoria and the Board of Aldermen, 26 June 1944. Rudy, *For Such a Time as This*, 116, 153–4. Rudy sees this notion of "home" as the philosophical basis for Ontario's 1949 Homes for Aged Act.

46 BCLL, Harvey, "Study of Chronic Diseases," 21.

47 BCA, GR 496, Box 23, File 12, "Annual Report of the Provincial Infirmary for the year ending March 31, 1942" and "Annual Report of the Provincial Infirmary for the year ending March 31, 1943."

48 RMC, Minute Book of the Aged Women's Home started May 1944, "44th Annual Report," 6 May 1952.

49 Means and Smith, *From Poor Law to Community Care*, 18; Rudy, *For Such a Time as This*, 153.

50 Guest, "Taylor Manor," 20.

51 Details from the provincial institutions were taken from BCA, GR 131, Box 2, File 12, "Annual Report, Provincial Home," 1 April 1950 to 31 March 1951; GR 496, Box 23, File 12, "Annual Report of the Provincial Infirmary for the year ending March 31, 1944," "Annual Report of the Provincial Infirmary for the year ending March 31, 1941," and "Annual Report of the Provincial Infirmary for the year ending March 31, 1943."

52 "The Salvation Army Matson Lodge," *Royal Architectural Institute of Canada Journal*, ser. 444, vol. 39, no. 8 (August 1962): 35–7.

53 See McFarland, "The Care of the Chronically Ill," for a discussion of chronic illness in the B.C. context. The American doctor Ernest Boas was a guru for McFarland and others interested in chronic disease at this time. See Boas, *The Unseen Plague*. The earliest Canadian study of this topic is likely the 1941 Special Committee of Montreal Social Workers, *The Case of the Chronically Ill in Montreal*. The 1946 Kellogg Foundation survey of hospitals in the province argued that chronic care patients were "cluttering up beds." BCA, GR 277, Box 2, File 2, "Graham Davis Report Concerning Health Care in B.C," 1946.

54 Graebner, *A History of Retirement*, 215–41. These ideas are discussed in a more contemporary context by Clough, *Old Age Homes*, 4–13, 176. For examples of professional writing on the subject by Canadians see Calder, "A Prescription for Longevity"; Tysoe, "An Integrated Community Programme"; and Bishop, "Edmonton's Friendship Club." For recreation for seniors in the United States see Achenbaum, *Shades of Grey*, 69. For Britain see Jerrome, "Me Darby, You Joan!"

55 Du Moulin, "Gordon House Serves Its Senior Citizens"; "Report of the Social Welfare Branch, 1947–48," SP, vol.1, 1949, P-62–63.

56 See "Annual Report of the Social Welfare Branch of the Department of Health and Social Welfare, 1950," SP, vol. 2, 1951, R-65; BCA, GR 496, Box 49, File 5 "Annual Report, Welfare Institutions Board, 1941."

57 BCA, GR 496, Box 49, File 5, "Annual Report, Welfare Institutions Board, 1941."

58 BCA, GR 678, Box 10, File 25, E. Pringle, "The Need for Chronic Disease Hospitals," 1953.

59 There is a huge body of documentation relating to this topic. For example, NA, RG 29, Vol. 909, File 479–316, Community Chest and Council of Greater Vancouver, "Report of the Special Committee Studying the Inadequacies of the Hospital Facilities for the Chronically Ill in the Vancouver Area," circa 1950s; Walker, "Better Provision Needed for the Chronically Ill"; Ward, "How Much Hospitalization is Really Necessary for the Chronically Ill?"; BCA, GR 277, Box 2, File 2, "Graham Davis Report Concerning Health Care in B.C," 1948; GR 678, Box 10, File 25, E. Pringle, "The Need for Chronic Disease Hospitals," 1953.

60 BCLL, Harvey, "Study of Chronic Diseases," 10, 15; BCA, GR 496, Box 23, File 12, M. Law, "Report of the Provincial Infirmary for the year ending March 31, 1945"; Box 23, File 12, M. Law, "Annual Report of the Provincial Infirmary for the year ending March 31, 1946"; GR 277, Box 5, File 1, M. Law, "Report on Provincial Infirmaries, 1950."

61 BCA, Add. MSS. 2818, File 27, Local Council of Women, Victoria, Temporary Committee to the Mayor of Victoria and the Board of

Aldermen, 26 June 1944; Gorge Road Hospital Papers, Gayton, "Gorge Road Hospital History, 1944 to 1977."

62 "Annual Report of the Welfare Institutions Licensing Board, 1949," *SP*, vol. 2, 1951, R-105.

63 Earl Eubank, Emory S. Bogardus, and Morton Deutsch were important theorists in this regard.

64 BCA, GR 131, Box 2, File 17, "Annual Report, Provincial Home, April 1, 1955 to March 31." Cassidy stated in 1938 that "entertainment and recreation ... would make them [the inmates] happier and more amenable to discipline." BCA, GR 496, Box 47, File 8, H. Cassidy, "Report on the Home for Incurables," 25 January 1938.

65 Details of various recreational activities taken from the following sources: BCA, GR 131, Box 2, File 17, "Annual Report, Provincial Home, April 1, 1955 to March 31"; GR 496, Box 23, File 12, "Annual Report of the Provincial Infirmary for the year ending March 31, 1942"; Guest, "Taylor Manor," 24; SSAA, Mount Saint Mary's Chronicles, 1950–51, 4.

66 The volunteer is also inevitably a "she." For example, Talker, "Services for Married Couples," 65.

67 Hill, "Old People Have a Future."

68 "Annual Report of the Social Welfare Branch for the Department of Health and Welfare, 1949," *SP*, vol. 2, 1950, R-88.

69 MacQuarrie, "The Care of An Ageing and Disabled Group," 16.

70 See, for example, Rowe et al., "The Care of the Chronically Ill," and Johnson, "Old Age: A Public Health Problem." For analysis of this in the American context see Achenbaum, *Shades of Grey*, 15.

71 Means and Smith, *From Poor Law to Community Care*, 219–21.

72 Lillian Martin, a pioneering American psychotherapist who specialized first in children and then in the elderly, found this in her early work on disturbed young people. Cited in Thane, "Geriatrics." For examples of negative attitudes toward the aged that explicitly or implicitly favoured institutionalization see Young, "Growing Old Gracefully," and "Annual Report of the Social Welfare Branch of the Department of Health and Welfare, 1950," *SP*, vol. 2, 1951, R-6.

73 Talker, "Services for Married Couples," 2–4, 13.

74 Achenbaum, *Shades of Grey*, 71.

75 BCA, GR 277, Box 7, File 4, A. Mann, "Report concerning a social worker for the Provincial Infirmary," 25 November 1952.

76 Rowe et al., "The Care of the Chronically Ill," and Barker, "On the Care of the Aged." For a description of the ideal components of community recreation for seniors from a B.C. perspective, see Talker, "Services for Married Couples," 58–61.

77 Graebner has a good analysis of group work theory and old age. "The Golden Age Clubs," 416–28. Talker, in her thesis on married couples

on social assistance, characterizes good adjustment as sociability, church attendance, and family connections. "Services for Married Couples," 26.

78 Clough, *Old Age Homes*, 158–9.

79 Guest, "Taylor Manor," 24.

80 BCA, GR 496, Box 49, File 5, "Annual Report, Welfare Institutions Board, 1942."

81 BCA, GR 277, Box 5, File 1, M. Law, "Report on the Provincial Infirmary, December 1948." These items were made by Allco residents in 1945. BCA, GR 496, Box 15, File 9, "Statement – February to November – Occupational Therapy," 12 December 1945. Harvey found that patients at Marpole were more content than those at Mount St Mary's, and used that information to critique the Sisters of Saint Ann for not providing occupational therapy for patients. BCLL, Harvey, "Study of Chronic Diseases," 15.

82 McFarland makes the perceptive observation that many elderly people equated social workers with relief investigators. "The Care of the Chronically Ill," 146.

83 Starr, *The Social Transformation*, 20.

84 RMC, Minute Book of the Aged Women's Home started May 1944, minutes of meeting, 2 December 1947.

85 BCA, GR 277, Box 7, File 3, F.B. Williscroft and J.A. McNab, "Characteristics of the Infirmary Service."

86 BCA, GR 678, Box 1, File 6, Lloyd Detwiller, "Review of Proposed New Chronic Treatment and Convalescent Coverage Program in British Columbia."

87 BCA, GR 277, Box 3, File 4, No author, confidential report, 26 August 1955; McFarland, "The Care of the Chronically Ill," 64, 143.

CHAPTER FOUR

1 Contemporary research has shown, not surprisingly, that entering residential accommodation is much more traumatic if the "environmental discontinuity" is greater. Tobin and Lieberman, *Last Home for the Aged*, 20.

2 My analysis of power among people we tend to see as powerless has been usefully informed by Janeway, *Powers of the Weak*.

3 Crowther found that the gender shift occurred around 1930, with increasing numbers of old women entering from 1921. *The Workhouse System*, 234–5. In a study of a Scottish residential home, it was found that by 1980 women outnumbered men 4.3:1. Kayser-Jones, *Old, Alone, and Neglected*, 56.

4 BCLL, Harvey, "Study of Chronic Diseases," 15.

5 VANCA, *City Reports*, "Report of Old People's Home, 1915," 27.

6 BCA, GR 496, Box 47, File 9, Zella Collins, "Report Prepared for the Advisory Board, Provincial Infirmary, 16–3–39"; BCLL, Harvey, "Study of Chronic Diseases."

7 Leydier, "Boarding Home Care for the Aged," 47.

8 Katz, *Poverty and Policy*, 126; Townsend, *The Last Refuge*, 55. Stewart found that of the men that entered Wellington County House of Industry between 1877 and 1907 90 per cent were working class and 70 per cent were unskilled labourers. "The Elderly Poor," 224.

9 The following inmate numbers were selected for analysis, spanning the admission years 1895–1965: 1–99, 300–399, 600–699, 900–999, 1,200–1,299, 1,500–1,599, 1,800–1,899. BCA, GR 131, Box 1, Vol. 1. These locations are a sample of those listed in the 1935–36 "Annual Report of the Provincial Home," BCA, GR 496, Box 29, File 2.

10 Other blue-collar occupations listed included teamster, bricklayer, longshoreman, expressman, and engineer. Non blue-collar occupations included photographer, architect, clerk, teacher, and journalist. Occupations that may have been replaced by mechanized modes of production included tanner, laceworker, axe-maker, and textile artist. Inmate statistics from the Old Men's Home are culled from patients' applications of the period. VCA-CR.

11 BCA, GR 678, Box 5, File 15, "Report on Visits to the Marpole and Allco Infirmaries, Feb 13th and 14th, 1958."

12 RMC, Minute Book for Home for Aged and Infirm Women beginning April 1901, minutes of meeting, 4 October 1907, and Minute Book for Aged and Infirm Woman's Home commencing April 1908, minutes of meeting, 6 Sept 1909.

13 This was also the case in Ottawa's Protestant Home for the Aged in the late nineteenth century, where younger men moved in temporarily during periods of illness or unemployment. Cook, "'A Quiet Place … to Die,'" 29. As late as 1960 in England and Wales younger, blind epileptic patients lived alongside the aged poor in former public assistance institutions, and unmarried mothers with their babies and homeless families found temporary accommodation. Townsend, *The Last Refuge*, 72.

14 VCA-CR, Box 22, File 4, Minutes of a Meeting of the Health (Special) Committee, 31 August 1933.

15 BCLL, Harvey, "Study of Chronic Diseases."

16 BCA, GR 496, Box 49, File 5, "Report Regarding the Administration of Welfare Institutions Act for the year ending December 31, 1942," table 2.

17 Residential statistics listed in this paragraph come from the following sources: BCLL, Harvey, "Study of Chronic Diseases"; BCA, GR 496, Box 49, File 5, "Report Regarding the Administration of Welfare

Institutions Act for the year ending December 31, 1942," table 2; McFarland, "The Care of the Chronically Ill," 67, appendix B, table L; VCA-CR.

18 VCA, *City Reports*, "Report of the Manager of the Home for Aged and Infirm, January 1908" and "Report of Manager of Home for the Aged and Infirm, January 1913."

19 BCA, GR 289, Box 4, File 3, Sub-Agent, Wilmer to P. Walker, 20 April 1925. Stewart makes this same point in reference to Wellington County House of Industry. "The Elderly Poor," 231. Crowther discusses English working-class hatred for the workhouse. *The Workhouse System*, ch. 2.

20 BCLL, Harvey, "Study of Chronic Diseases"; BCA, GR 277, Box 5, File 2, Memo by H.P. Bell, 9 May 1955.

21 It is not certain how long the Chinese Old Man's Home of New Westminster remained in operation nor how many residents it had. BCA, GR 1582, B.C. Register of Companies, Box 182, File 376.

22 "Dream Home for Old Folks," *Province*, 26 February 1944; "Where old people are understood," 29; Guest, "Taylor Manor," 9.

23 BCA, GR 738, "Report and Evidence concerning Commission of Inquiry into the Provincial Home, Kamloops, 1903–04."

24 VCA-CR, Box 5, File 2, and Box 5, File 5. An application was turned down because the man was an invalid, and another inmate with heart disease and dropsy was removed to hospital.

25 Ibid., Box 28, File 3, G. Havard to Alderman F.A. Willis and Home Committee, 15 July 1943.

26 This was not the case at Taylor Manor, where administrators were trying to transform the institution from "a workhouse to a boarding home." Residents who were ill for any length of time were moved to a nursing home. Guest, "Taylor Manor," 30.

27 BCA, GR 277, Box 3, File 3, M. Law, "Annual Report of the Provincial Infirmary," 1956.

28 BCLL, Harvey, "Study of Chronic Diseases," 16, 19.

29 Snell, "The First Grey Lobby," 3.

30 VCA-CR, Box 24, File 5, June 1938, letter from G. Havard to Alderman Okell; VCA-CR, Box 25, File 1, "Superintendent's Report," 20 January 1939.

31 Haber, *Beyond Sixty-Five*, 87.

32 City of Victoria, No. 3018, A By-law Relating to the Operation and Maintenance of a Home for Aged and Infirm Men; Guest, "Taylor Manor," 27.

33 VCA-CR, Box 16, File 4, "Report of the Home Committee," 11 May 1920.

34 SMA, Clerk's Department, Box 87, File 3, 1946 letter from John Tribe, Municipal Clerk to Wilfred Greene, City Treasurer of New Westminster.

35 In 1950 the per diem at the Provincial Infirmary was $1.50. BCA, GR 277, Box 5, File 1, I.R. Buckley to A.W.E. Pitkethley, 17 October 1950; A.D. Turnbull to Lloyd Detwiller, 2 November 1950.

36 RMC, Minute Book for Home for Aged and Infirm Women beginning April 1901, special meeting, 18 May 1907.

37 Ibid., minutes of meeting, 6 July 1915.

38 For a contemporary discussion of depersonalization and routinized care in old age homes see Kayser-Jones, *Old, Alone, and Neglected*, 43. Regimented daily schedules were customary at poor law institutions for the aged in other parts of Canada. Stewart, "The Elderly Poor," 232–3.

39 This schedule is based on an early report, but it is reasonable to assume that a similar program would have been followed in later years. VCA, *City Reports*, "Report on Home for Aged and Infirm," 31 December 1893.

40 RMC, Minute Book for Home for Aged and Infirm Women beginning April 1901, minutes of meeting, 4 February 1907; Rose Manor Minute Book, 1917–1926, minutes of meeting, 17 October 1916.

41 Leydier, "Boarding Home Care for the Aged," 128–9. Bathing was traditionally a weekly event at English workhouses, where elderly people were afforded no personal privacy during the process. Crowther, *The Workhouse System*, 196, and Townsend, *The Last Refuge*, 91–2.

42 VCA-CR, Box 16, File 16, "Committee Report," 14 March 1921. The process of discarding clothes from the "old life" and replacing them with institutional attire was a common practice in all kinds of public institutions, including prisons and asylums. In England and Wales individual clothing was taken away and inmates given garments, perhaps with the name of the institution and the number of the ward or blocked marked on it. These garments, used but clean, would of course have been previously worn by inmates now deceased. Townsend, *The Last Refuge*, 90.

43 VCA-CR, Box 22, File 4, Minutes of a Meeting of the Health (Special) Committee, 31 August 1933.

44 BCA, GR 277, Box 5, File 1, M. Law to A.W.E. Pitkethley, 6 August 1951.

45 BCA, GR 496, Box 12, File 1, "Rules and Regulations for the Government of the Provincial Home," 25 July 1895.

46 RMC, Minute Book for Home for Aged and Infirm Women beginning April 1901, special meeting, 21 May 1904.

47 RMC, Minute Book for Aged and Infirm Woman's Home commencing April 1908, minutes of meeting, 7 February 1910.

48 Ibid., minutes of meeting, 29 November 1909.

49 RMC, Minute Book of the Aged Women's Home started May 5, 1936, minutes of meeting, 1 April 1941.

50 See Stewart, "The Elderly Poor," for a description of workhouse regulations.

51 VCA-CR, Box 2, File 2, "Home for Aged and Infirm Committee's Report," 28 October 1892. BCA, GR 496, Box 12, File 1, "Rules and Regulations for the Government of the Provincial Home," 25 July 1895.

52 The 1912 report stated, "in fact it has been a very harmonious year among the inmates, there being no call for the patrol wagon." VCA, *City Reports*, "Report of the Manager of the Home for Aged and Infirm," 5 January 1912.

53 Struthers, *The Limits of Affluence*, 56–7, and Snell, *The Citizen's Wage*, 48.

54 BCA, GR 738, "Report and Evidence concerning Commission of Inquiry into the Provincial Home, Kamloops, 1903–04," 32.

55 Ibid., 34.

56 Gubrium notes the central role of food in the lives of residents of old age homes. *Living and Dying at Murray Manor*, 172–5. See also Crowther, *The Workhouse System*, 213–19.

57 RMC, Minute book for Aged and Infirm Women's Home commencing April 1908, minutes of meeting, 6 October 1914.

58 Ibid, minutes of meeting, 1 August 1916.

59 RMC, Minute Book for Home for Aged and Infirm Women beginning January 1917, minutes of meeting held 9 March 1918.

60 Goffman, *Asylums*, 43–124.

61 Crowther provides an excellent discussion of the philosophies and practices of workhouse labour. *The Workhouse System*, 196–201.

62 VCA, *City Reports*, "Report of Home for Aged and Infirm, for Year ending December 31, 1894." *City Reports*, "Report of the Home Manager," 17 March 1920; VCA-CR, Box 18, File 3, "Report of the Home Committee," 21 July 1924.

63 BCA, GR 738, "Report and Evidence concerning Commission of Inquiry into the Provincial Home, Kamloops, 1903–04," 36, 38.

64 BCA, GR 131, Box 3, Envelope M, A. Noble to relative, 19 July 1923 and 10 August 1923.

65 VCA-CR, Box 18, File 5, "Home for Aged and Infirm Committee Report," 9 March 1925.

66 BCA, GR 738, "Report and Evidence concerning Commission of Inquiry into the Provincial Home, Kamloops, 1903–04," 49.

67 BCA, GR 131, Box 3, Envelope T, A. Noble to P. Walker, 29 September 1936.

68 RMC, Minute Book for Aged and Infirm Woman's Home commencing April 1908, minutes of meeting, 3 June 1913.

69 OB-DHM, 5–6

70 BCA, GR 131, Box 3, File 1, A. Noble to P. Walker, 29 October 1936.

71 Guest, "Taylor Manor," 29.

72 "Matron Retires From Home," *Victoria Daily Times*, 28 February 1947.

73 The memoirs of David Havard contain descriptions of a number of inmates. The authenticity of Havard's recollections is borne out by the applications for admission to the Home that match the descriptions of Havard's fruit peddler and scissor grinder. OB-DHM, 4–5.

74 BCA, GR 738, "Report and Evidence concerning Commission of Inquiry into the Provincial Home, Kamloops, 1903–04," 32.

75 BCA, GR 131, Box 3, Envelope T, Superintendent, Provincial Home to Deputy Provincial Secretary, 9 September 1922.

76 VANCA, *City Reports*, Annual Reports, Old People's Home, 1920–1939.

77 BCA, GR 738, "Report and Evidence concerning Commission of Inquiry into the Provincial Home, Kamloops, 1903–04."

78 BCA, GR 277, Box 5, File 1, D. Turnbull, "Memo of Visit to Infirmaries on July 19, 1950," 21 July 1950.

79 Townsend makes this point in *The Last Refuge*, 340–1. Crowther found that, even well into the twentieth century, inmate labour was irrevocably associated with the idea of punishment. *The Workhouse System*, 201.

80 BCA, GR 907, Harold Bird, "Commissioners Report on the Home of the Friendless," 1937, 11.

81 "Soroptimist House Friendly Haven for Retired Women," *News Herald*, 2 April 1947, 7.

82 RMC, Minute Book for Home for Aged and Infirm Women beginning April 1901, minutes of meeting, 4 March 1907; Minute Book for Home for Aged and Infirm Women beginning April 1908, minutes of meeting, 28 March 1910; minutes of meeting, 10 March 1916.

83 Other Canadian historians have found seasonal patterns of male discharge and recommittal at old age institutions. Stewart, "The Elderly Poor," 225–6, and Cook, "'A Quiet Place ... to Die,'" 29.

84 This point is based on patient movements detailed in three annual reports of the Provincial Home: BCA, GR 496, Box 29, File 2, "Annual Report, Provincial Home, Kamloops, for the Year ending March 31, 1936"; GR 131, Box 2, File 2, "Annual Report, Provincial Home, Kamloops, Fiscal Year ending March 31, 1941"; File 12, "Annual Report, Provincial Home, Kamloops, Fiscal Year April 1st, 1950 to March 31st, 1951."

85 BCA, GR 131, Box 3, File 2, B.C. Provincial Police Report, 9 November 1923.

86 Ibid., Envelope R, Police Constable, Vernon to Deputy Provincial Secretary, 21 July 1924.

87 Ibid., J.H. to A. Noble, 27 August 1928.

88 Ibid., Envelope F, letters from the Superintendent, Provincial Home to Deputy Provincial Secretary, 29 July 1924, 1 September 1924, 18 July 1925, 16 September 1925, 4 October 1926.

89 Talker, "Services for Married Couples," 45.
90 Snell, *The Citizen's Wage*, 49. Stewart found that elderly women, although less likely to enter the House of Industry, were more likely to remain lengthy periods and die in the institution. "The Elderly Poor," 228–31.
91 RMC, Minute Book for Home for Aged and Infirm Women beginning April 1901, minutes of meeting, 2 March 1903; Minute Book for Home for Aged and Infirm Women commencing April 1908, minutes of meeting, 5 August 1913; Minute Book for Home for Aged and Infirm Women commencing January 1917, minutes of meeting, 3 December 1918.
92 RMC, Minute Book for Home for Aged and Infirm Women beginning April 1901, minutes of meeting, 3 September 1901; minutes of meeting, 1 April 1907; Minute Book for Aged and Infirm Women Home commencing April 1908, minutes of meeting, 3 October 1910.
93 Current studies of residential accommodation for the aged have emphasized the importance that residents place on "stepping out" from the institution. Gubrium, *Living and Dying at Murray Manor*, 84.
94 RMC, Minute Book starting May 1944, minutes of meeting, 8 July 1952.
95 BCA, GR 277, Box 7, File 6, patient letter, 21 June 1954.
96 Ibid., File 2, M. Law to A.W.E. Pitkethley, 6 December 1952.
97 Ibid., Box 3, File 4, no author, untitled confidential report, 26 August 1955.
98 McFarland, "The Care of the Chronically Ill," 79, and Leydier, "Boarding Home Care for the Aged," 111.
99 Studies cited in Tobin and Lieberman, *Last Home for the Aged*, 9–10. See also Townsend, *The Last Refuge*, 341–2 and Crowther, *The Workhouse System*, 213.
100 BCA, GR 277, Box 5, File 1, D. Turnbull, "Memo of Visit to Infirmaries on July 19, 1950," 21 July 1950.
101 BCLL, Harvey, "Study of Chronic Diseases," 12, 15, 22.
102 BCA, GR 738, "Report and Evidence concerning Commission of Inquiry into the Provincial Home, Kamloops, 1903–04," 27, 35.
103 RMC, Minute Book for Home for Aged and Infirm Women beginning January 1917, minutes of meeting, 7 January 1919.
104 VANCA, Series 452, 106-F1, File 3, Vancouver Old People's Home, Daily Book, January 1917.
105 Leydier, "Boarding Home Care for the Aged," 80.
106 RMC, Minute Book for Aged and Infirm Women's Home commencing April 1908, minutes of meeting, 2 August 1909, and Minute Book for Aged and Infirm Women's Home beginning May 1944, minutes of meeting, 3 February 1948.
107 BCLL, Harvey, "Study of Chronic Diseases," 21. Gubrium also notes the central role that food plays in patients' lives at old age homes. *Living and Dying at Murray Manor*, 172–5.

108 References for this paragraph come from the following sources: RMC, Minute Book for Home for Aged and Infirm Women commencing April 1908, minutes of special meeting, 13 February 1910; minutes of meeting, 4 June 1912; minutes of meeting, 31 December 1912 and special meeting, 23 January 1913 and minutes of meeting, 30 June 1913; Minute Book for Home for Aged and Infirm Women beginning January 1917, minutes of meeting, 6 February 1923.

109 BCA, GR 738, "Report and Evidence concerning Commission of Inquiry into the Provincial Home, Kamloops, 1903–04," 34.

110 McFarland, "The Care of the Chronically Ill," 79.

111 For example, on 2 February 1917 inmates returned to the Old People's Home intoxicated. VANCA, Series 452, 106-F1, File 3, Vancouver Old People's Home, Daily Book, February 1917.

112 BCA, GR 277, Box 3, File 4, no author, untitled confidential report, 26 August 1955.

113 Women's Home references from the following sources: RMC, Minute Book for Home for Aged and Infirm Women beginning April 1901, minutes of meeting, 29 February 1904; minutes of meeting, 9 January 1905; Minute Book for Home for Aged and Infirm Women commencing April 1908, minutes of a special meeting, 20 January 1909.

114 RMC, Minute Book for Home for Aged and Infirm Women commencing April 1908, minutes of meeting, 5 December 1910.

115 RMC, Minute Book for Home for Aged and Infirm Women beginning January 1917, minutes of meeting, 6 May 1919.

116 VCA-CR, Box 22, File 4, Minutes of a Meeting of the Health (Special) Committee, 31 August 1933.

117 The old people I talk about did not have effective avenues to those in power like Krasnick Warsh's middle-class mental health patients, or the senior citizen activists that Snell describes. Krasnick Warsh, *Moments of Unreason*, 120, 133–41, and Snell, "The First Grey Lobby."

118 Townsend, *The Last Refuge*, 94.

119 Tobin and Lieberman cite studies that found that residents in old age homes feel personally insignificant and impotent, view themselves as old, docile, and submissive, and live in the past rather than the future. *Last Home for the Aged*, 9–10.

120 VANCA, Series 452, 106-F1, File 3, Vancouver Old People's Home, Daily Book.

121 VCA, *City Reports*, "Report of the Manager of the Home for Aged and Infirm," 11 January 1904.

122 RMC, Minute Book for Home for Aged and Infirm Women beginning April 1901, minutes of meeting, 4 March 1907.

123 BCA, GR 131, Box 3, Envelope Mc, Superintendent, Provincial Home to J.M., 19 August 1927.

124 OB-DHM, 3.

125 VCA-CR, Box 28, File 5, "Old Men's Home Annual Report," 1943.

126 BCA, GR 496, Box 47, File 9, Zella Collins, "Report Prepared for Advisory Board, Provincial Infirmary, March 16, 1939."

127 Ibid.

128 BCA, GR 277, Box 5, File 1, M. Law, "Report of the Provincial Infirmary, December 1948."

129 Townsend, *The Last Refuge*, 95.

130 Studies of old age homes have found the general attitude of institutionalized aged toward death to be one of acceptance. Gubrium, *Living and Dying at Murray Manor*, 204, and Townsend, *The Last Refuge*, 96.

131 Coates, "Death in British Columbia," 40–5.

132 See Kayser-Jones, *Old, Alone, and Neglected*, 49–51.

133 RMC, Minute Book for Aged and Infirm Woman's Home commencing April 1908, minutes of meeting, 30 June 1913.

134 RMC, Minute Book for Aged and Infirm Woman's Home commencing January 1917, minutes of meeting, 1 October 1918.

135 SSAA, MSM Collection, RG 43, Box 4, File 3, E.G. to Sister Superior Mary Patrick, 8 March 1958.

136 McFarland, "The Care of the Chronically Ill," 64, 143.

137 BCLL, Harvey, "Study of Chronic Diseases," and BCA, GR 277, Box 3, File 4, confidential report, no author, 26 August 1955.

138 Berton, "25 Pensioners Happy at Mother Fowler's," 13.

139 BCLL, Harvey, "Study of Chronic Diseases," 18.

140 Struthers, *The Limits of Affluence*, 57–8.

141 Rothman, *The Discovery of the Asylum*, 42–3.

142 BCA, Photo Collection, Maynard Files, G. Havard to A.M., 7 November 1928.

143 OB-DHM, 5–7.

144 BCA, GR 131, Box 3, Envelope T, Noble to relatives, 31 March 1937.

145 Townsend makes this point as well. *The Last Refuge*, 92.

146 Townsend concluded that more than two-fifths of head staff were unnecessarily authoritarian in their dealings with residents and that matrons held too rigidly to the medical model and professional standards, sometimes at the cost of compassionate care for the aged. *The Last Refuge*, 84–9.

147 VCA-CR, Box 22, File 4, Minutes of a Meeting of the Health (Special) Committee, 31 August 1933.

148 RMC, Minute book for Aged and Infirm Women's Home commencing April 1908, minutes of meeting, 3 February 1914.

149 Ibid., 2 December 1913.

150 VCA-CR, Box 22, File 4, Minutes of a Meeting of the Health (Special) Committee, 31 August 1933.

151 Leydier, "Boarding Home Care for the Aged," 118–21.

152 References for this paragraph come from RMC, Minute Book for Home for Aged and Infirm Women beginning April 1901, minutes of meeting, 23 April 1901; Minute book for Aged and Infirm Women's Home commencing April 1908, minutes of meeting, 2 December 1913; 6 August 1918; Minute Book for Home for Aged and Infirm Women beginning April 1901, minutes of meeting, 6 February 1905; 7 January 1907.

153 RMC, Rose Manor Minute Book, 1917–1926, minutes of meeting, 6 April 1920; 5 July 1920; 3 July 1923.

154 References for this paragraph come from ibid., 5 October 1920; 6 May 1924.

155 References for this paragraph come from RMC, Minute book for Aged and Infirm Women's Home commencing April 1908, minutes of meeting, 4 September 1914; 3 June 1919; and RMC, Rose Manor Minute Book, 1917–1926, minutes of meeting, 4 June 1918; Minute book for Aged and Infirm Women's Home commencing April 1908, minutes of meeting, 15 February 1916; 5 August 1913.

156 RMC, Minute book for Aged and Infirm Women's Home commencing April 1908, minutes of meeting, 3 April 1909, 5 December 1916.

157 RMC, Rose Manor Minute Book, 1917–1926, minutes of meeting, 7 August 1923; Minute Book of the Aged Women's Home started May 1944, minutes of meeting, 1 April 1947, 4 March and 1 April 1952.

158 RMC, Rose Manor Minute Book, 1917–1926, minutes of meeting, 2 July 1919.

159 RMC, Minute Book of the Aged Women's Home started 5 May 1936, minutes of meeting, 5 September 1939.

160 RMC, Rose Manor Minute Book, 1917–1926, minutes of meeting, 5 December 1922.

161 RMC, Minute Book of the Aged Women's Home started 5 May 1936, minutes of meeting, 1 February 1938.

162 OB-DHM, 2.

163 Leydier, "Boarding Home Care for the Aged," 65, 67.

164 "95-Yr-Old Hannah Stainer Will Be Life of Old Ladies' Christmas Party," newsclipping in RMC, Minute Book beginning May 1944, final page in volume.

165 BCA, GR 277, Box 5, File 1, D. Turnbull, "Memo of Visit to Infirmaries on July 19, 1950," 21 July 1950.

166 Thompson and Golden, *The Hospital*, 271.

167 BCA, GR 496, Box 23, File 12, "Report of the Provincial Infirmary, Marpole, for the year ending March 31, 1941"; BCLL, Harvey, "Study of Chronic Diseases," 11.

168 "Allco and Marpole," *Province*, 29 January 1947, 4.

169 BCA, GR 496, Box 47, File 8, H. Cassidy, "Report on the Home for Incurables," 25 January 1938.

170 "Residents Object to New Home," *Vancouver Sun*, 18 May 1943, 12.

171 SMA, Clerk's Department, Box 71, File 5, J. Nixon to W. Green, 1943.

172 VANCA, Series 452, 106-FI, File 3, Vancouver Old People's Home, Daily Book, 11 March 1917.

173 VCA-CR, Box 29, File 3, H.C.F. Reston to G. Havard, 26 October 1944, and G. Havard to F.A. Willis, 26 October 1944.

174 RMC, Minute Book for Home for Aged and Infirm Women beginning April 1901, minutes of meeting, 2 November 1903.

175 VCA-CR, Box 29, File 3, G. Havard to F.A. Willis, 26 October 1944.

176 RMC, Minute Book of Aged and Infirm Women's Home beginning January 1917, news clipping from local paper, 1919; minutes of meeting, 7 October 1919; Minute Book of the Aged Women's Home started 5 May 1936, minutes of board meeting, 4 July 1939.

177 RMC, James Morton, "To my Neighbours of the Aged Women's Home," 1942.

178 OB-DHM, 7.

179 VCA, *City Reports*, "Report on Home for Aged and Infirm, 1893."

180 VCA-CR, Box 24, File 5, "Report of the Home Committee," 16 May 1938.

181 SSAA, "Chronicles: Mount St Mary, 1949–1950."

182 VCA, *City Reports*, "Home for Aged and Infirm Manager's Report, 7 January 1898."

183 BCA, GR 496, Box 23, File 12, C.M. Motherwell, "Annual Report of the Provincial Infirmary for the year ending March 31, 1943"; C.M. Motherwell, "Annual Report of the Provincial Infirmary for the year ending March 31, 1944"; and C.M. Motherwell, "Annual Report of the Provincial Infirmary for the year ending March 31, 1945."

184 RMC, Minute Book of the Aged Women's Home started 5 May 1936, minutes of board meeting, 3 January 1939.

185 VANCA, Series 452, 106-FI, File 3, Vancouver Old People's Home, Daily Book, December 1917 and January 1918.

186 Ibid., 6 July 1917.

187 BCA, GR 277, Box 5, File 1, M. Law, "Report of the Provincial Infirmary, December 1948."

188 BCA, GR 496, Box 23, File 12, C. M. Motherwell, "Annual Report of the Provincial Infirmary for the year ending March 31, 1945," and GR 277, Box 5, File 1, M. Law, "Report of the Provincial Infirmary, December 1950."

189 BCA, GR 131, Box 3, Envelope R, Superintendent to relative, 27 September 1928.

190 VCA-CR, Box 16, File 5, "Report of the Home Committee," 9 May 1921.

CHAPTER FIVE

1 Novak, *Aging and Society*, chs 8 and 11.
2 For example, the Quick Response Team, a program developed by Victoria's Capital Regional District to support older people in their homes after illness or accidents. Cited in ibid., 208–9.
3 Means and Smith are an exception to a general trend within policy analysis of ignoring history. The two authors explore these ideas in *From Poor Law to Community Care*, 3.
4 Historians have singled out Weir as Pattullo's strongest ally within the provincial cabinet regarding reform issues. See Fisher, *Duff Pattullo*, 233, 250–1, and Ormsby, *British Columbia: A History*, 456–7. For a discussion of public health policy in B.C. during the 1930s and early 1940s see Davies, "Competent Professionals and Modern Methods."
5 Moffatt, *A Poetics of Social Work*.
6 Although there has not been enough detailed historical analysis of health and social welfare programs during the Depression to say that B.C. was exceptional in this regard, this kind of optimistic expansion was only matched by Quebec. Elsewhere, retrenchment was typical. In Ontario, for example, after Mitch Hepburn's 1934 election victory, the incoming welfare minister, David Croll, fired all eleven provincial pension inspectors and disbanded local pension boards in all but four Ontario cities. Struthers, "Regulating the Elderly," 18.
7 This interpretation of corporatism and the role of the expert in the corporate state is based on the ideas of Harold Perkin. See Perkin, *The Rise of Professional Society*, ch. 8.
8 See Achenbaum, *Crossing Frontiers*, especially ch. 2.
9 My approach here is based on the thesis that professionals within state bureaucracy are active agents with their own policy agendas. The programs they develop naturally reflect their own professional allegiances. For a fuller development of this approach see Skocpol, *Protecting Soldiers and Mothers*, 1–62.
10 Quadagno has published extensively on the American state and pensions. See Quadagno and Harrington-Meyer, "Organized Labor," 181–96, and Quadagno, *The Transformation of Old Age Security*. Also Graebner, *A History of Retirement*.
11 Achenbaum, *Shades of Grey*; Haber, *Beyond Sixty-Five*; Cole, *The Journey of Life*.
12 Leydier, "Boarding Home Care for the Aged," 34.
13 Rudy, *For Such a Time as This*, 135
14 See Webster, "The Elderly and the Early National Health Service," 165–93.

15 Cassidy devoted a section of his 1945 survey of Canadian health and welfare provision to B.C.'s Hospital Clearance plan. *Public Health and Welfare Reorganization*, 92–6. The clearances program was part of larger provincial hospital reforms that made local hospitals adopt standardized accounting and administration procedures. Pringle, "British Columbia Shows the Way."

16 Memos from Ward to Weir give a very cynical interpretation of this process, stating that hospitals had been used by families, physicians, and local authorities as "sump pits" for unwanted elderly. BCA, GR 496, Box 49, File 9, P. Ward to G. Weir, 11 January 1938.

17 Haber found the process of excluding old people from hospitals taking place in American hospitals at the turn of the century. *Beyond Sixty-Five*, 90–1.

18 Rosenberg, "Inward Vision and Outward Glance," 346–91. A similar process of patient selection was at work in British municipal hospitals during the inter-war years, the same period covered in this chapter. Means and Smith, *From Poor Law to Community Care*, 20.

19 BCA, GR 496, Box 49, File 9, P. Ward to G. Weir, 11 January 1938; H. Cassidy to G. Weir, 31 January 1938.

20 For the next decade Amyot worked his way up the public health ladder in B.C., becoming assistant provincial health officer and adviser on hospital services in 1936 and provincial health officer in 1940. He spent the years 1938–40 in the United States again, working as an administrative associate of the American Public Health Association and as a professor of public health administration at the University of Minnesota. Amyot's career details are taken from "Report of the Provincial Board of Health," 1940, SP, vol. 1, 1943, E7–8, "Deputy Minister to Retire," and a copy of his curriculum vitae.

21 The concept of man as a machine has been identified as the essence of the Rockefeller capitalist vision of health and is evident in a 1937 speech that Amyot made to the provincial branch of the Canadian Physical Education Association. Brown, *Rockefeller Medicine Men*, 116–22; VANCA, Clippings File, 22 December 1937.

22 Percy Ward was a First World War veteran who subsequently managed Burrard Wood and Fuel Company and was secretary of the Burrard Inlet Tunnel and Bridge Company. BCA, GR 496, Box 24, File 7, P. Ward to Amyot, 11 October 1936; "Funeral rites today for B.C.'s 'Mr Hospital,'" *Province*, 5 February 1964, 7; "Percy Ward Rites Today," *Vancouver Sun*, 5 February 1964, 20.

23 Amyot's survey has been lost. We are left with two interpretive reports, one in Province of British Columbia, *Hospital Statistics*, 1937, 5–6, the other an address titled "Hospital Control" that Amyot gave to the health and welfare staff in January 1937. The latter is located in the BCLL.

24 Documents covering this early clearance activity are located in: BCA, GR 496, Box 49, File 9, P. Ward to G. Weir, 11 January 1938; H. Cassidy to G. Weir, 31 January 1938; F. Mutrie, "Report on Hospital Clearance," 7 March 1938; VCA-CR, Box 24, File 4, D. Muire to J.A. Worthington, 18 February 1938.

25 BCLL, Amyot, "Hospital Control."

26 BCA, GR 496, Box 49, File 8, P. Ward to P. Walker, 2 June 1942. Cassidy argued in 1938 that hospital clearance cases could be cared for in infirmaries and boarding homes at a rate of $1 or $1.50 per day, while the per diem cost of maintaining a patient in an acute hospital bed was $3. File 9, H. Cassidy to G. Weir, 31 January 1938.

27 For a definition of New Liberalism see Perkin, *The Rise of Professional Society*, 140, and Freeden, *The New Liberalism*, 54–7, 256–7.

28 Cassidy went to the University of California and then on to the Brookings School of Economics and Government in Washington, where he received a Ph.D. in economics in 1926. UTA, B72–0022, Box 22, File 2, Allon Peebles, "Harry Morris Cassidy, 1900–1951."

29 Biographers have emphasized Cassidy's socialist or Fabian alliances, but Cassidy straddled the hazy ideological divide between the Fabians and New Liberalism. Irving, "Canadian Fabians," 7–28.

30 Holland was born in Nova Scotia and educated at Ryerson Public School and St Mildred's College in Toronto. She trained as a nurse at Montreal General Hospital and served in the war nursing service from 1915 to 1919. *Canadian Who's Who*, 1936, 518. She attended Simmons College from 1918 to 1920, taking courses in both the School of Social Work and the School of Household Economics. Simmons College Archives, *Simmons College Catalogue*, 1918–1919, 38 and *Simmons College Catalogue*, 1919–1920, 44.

31 BCA, GR 496, Box 49, File 8, P. Ward to P. Walker, 2 June 1942.

32 BCLL, Harvey, "The Generalized Social Worker." For a personal account of the working life of one of the first welfare fieldworkers, see Paulson, "East Kootenay Health and Welfare Service, 1936–1938."

33 UTA, B72–0022, Box 58, File 2, H. Cassidy to G. Weir, 6 September 1935. BCA, GR 496, Box 57, file 11, no author (likely Cassidy), memo, 19 December 1934.

34 BCA, GR 496, Box 49, File 9, P. Ward to all Welfare Visitors, Circular, 26 January 1938.

35 Ibid., Welfare Field Service Report, 26 January 1939.

36 The stated policy of both the Pattullo administration and the Coalition government from 1941 was to hire trained social workers whenever possible. Cassidy, "British Columbia Provincial Workers Meet," 48–50. See also "Public Welfare in British Columbia," 2–6.

37 Struthers, *The Limits of Affluence*, 150–2.

38 Fischer, *Growing Old in America*, and Cole, "The Spectre of Old Age," 23–37.

39 Ehrenreich, *The Altruistic Imagination*, 76–7. Brian Gratton argues that use of casework techniques fostered a focus on the individual and was one reason for the conservative philosophy of social workers during this period. "Social Workers and Old Age Pensions," 403–15. Charlotte Whitton, director of the Canadian Welfare Council from 1922 to 1941, is an excellent illustration of this trend in Canada. During the 1930s she repeatedly demanded that professional social workers be hired, to administer restrictive aid only to "legitimate" claimants. Struthers, "A Profession in Crisis," 114–15.

40 BCA, GR 496, Box 24, File 7, P. Ward to P. Walker, 14 June 1937; Box 49, File 9, P. Ward to all Welfare Visitors, Circular, 26 January 1938; Box 50, File 1, H. Cassidy to G. Weir, 1 March 1937.

41 For the City of Vancouver grant, BCA, GR 496, Box 50, File 1, H. Cassidy to G. Weir, 31 March 1938. For the City of Victoria grant, ibid., Box 49, File 9, H. Cassidy to G. Weir, 7 April 1938.

42 BCLL, Harvey, "The Generalized Social Worker."

43 "Describe Inmates of Home as Poorly Clad and Fearful," *Victoria Colonist*, 3 February 1937.

44 BCA, GR 496, Box 45, File 5, J. Marshall to G.M. Weir, 22 December 1938.

45 BCA, GR 911, British Columbia, "Report of the Commission of Welfare Institutions and Nursing Homes," 1938, 5.

46 Ibid., 9, 24.

47 Ibid. and GR 907, British Columbia, "Report and Evidence concerning the Home of the Friendless," 1937.

48 The most complete description of the scope and functioning of the Welfare Institutions Licensing Act and Board can be found in chapter 3 of Leydier, "Boarding Home Care for the Aged."

49 BCA, GR 496, Box 49, File 5, "Annual Report of the Welfare Institutions Board for the Calendar Year 1941," 4. For a discussion of B.C.'s kindergartens and the board see Weiss, "An Essential Year for the Child," 139–62.

50 BCA, GR 496, Box 49, File 5, "Annual Report of the Welfare Institutions Board for the Calendar Year 1942," 3. Because private hospitals were taking in increasing numbers of elderly patients during this period the Provincial Office of the Inspector of Hospitals was also dealing with growing numbers of aged in institutions.

51 BCA, GR 911, British Columbia, "Report of the Commission of Welfare Institutions and Nursing Homes," 1938, 12.

52 All information and quote from Leydier, "Boarding Home Care for the Aged," 36–9.

53 BCA, GR 496, Box 49, File 5, "Annual Report of the Chief Inspector, Welfare Institutions Licensing Act for the year ending April 1, 1939."

54 Ibid., Box 22, File 7, memo from E. Pringle to P. Ward, Inspector of Hospitals, 13 July 1944; Box 49, File 5, "Annual Report of the Welfare Institutions Board for the Calendar Year, 1941."

55 Province of British Columbia, *Hospital Statistics*, 1948, 7.

56 BCA, GR 496, Box 22, File 7, P. Ward to Norman Baker, 27 July 1944.

57 "News Notes," 69.

58 Page did most of the casework and Pringle the administrative tasks. BCA, GR 496, Box 49, File 5, "Annual Report of the Welfare Institutions Board for the Calendar Year, 1941."

59 The number of American women doing research in these areas from the 1930s is striking, and included Ruth Shonle Caven, Ethel Shandas, and Bernice L. Neugarten.

60 Other scholars have noted that civil servants tend to push for the advancement of the programs they are responsible for, as it enhances their own position. For example, Myles, "Comparative Public Policies for the Elderly," 34–5.

61 BCA, GR 496, Box 49, File 9, Report by F. Mutrie, 7 March 1938; Report by M.F. Hunter, 2 June 1938. Seven cases were not included in my calculations.

62 RMC, Minute Book of the Aged Women's Home started 5 May 1936, minutes of meeting, 3 May 1938.

63 Sources for Victoria hospital clearances: SSAA, Mount Saint Mary's Correspondence, G. Davidson to P. Walker, 12 August 1939; VCA-CR, Box 25, File 5, "Report of the Relief Committee," 8 January 1940; Box 27, File 2, "Report of the Health and Welfare Committee," 31 October 1941.

64 For illustrations of current community innovations for B.C.'s seniors see Social Planning and Research Council of B.C. and United Way Research Services, *The Learnings From the New Horizons, Partners in Aging Projects*.

65 Gordon, "The New Feminist Scholarship," 23.

66 Province of British Columbia, *Hospital Statistics*, 1945, 7.

67 See n70 in ch. 2 for examples of professional ageism.

68 UTA, B72–0022, Box 39, File 1, Interview with Amy Leigh, December 1943. Amy Leigh, then provincial assistant superintendent of welfare, reported that the relief men scorned the social work methods used by the women as "slack."

69 Cassidy, *Public Health and Welfare Reorganization*, 132–7.

70 Barman, *The West Beyond the West*, 275.

71 Crowther also makes this point for Britain in the inter-war period. Policy developments were ad hoc solutions to immediate problems

rather than planned programs like the hospital clearances in B.C. *British Social Policy*, 73–4.

72 As previously noted, in n8 of ch. 3, Snell discusses the development of the "senior citizen" – both the term and the concept – in Canada. Snell, *The Citizen's Wage*, introduction.

73 Analysis of resolutions presented at Social Credit conventions during its first five terms in government reveals a definite sympathy within the party for the aged who suffered financial hardship. Between 1950 and 1965 fourteen conference resolutions regarding housing and residential facilities for the aged and chronically ill were presented. In addition to resolutions concerning accommodation for the elderly, another thirty-two resolutions dealing with the elderly were presented at Social Credit conferences. Byron et al., "The Social Welfare Philosophy," 46, 57.

74 Barman, *The West Beyond the West*, 281.

75 Parker, *The Elderly and Residential Care*, 12.

76 Achenbaum, *Shades of Grey*, 40, and Achenbaum, *Old Age in the New Land*, 151.

77 In Britain, there was a dramatic shift under Thatcher from nearly complete dependence on public sector homes for the aged to private sector domination by 1989. Peace et al., *Re-evaluating Residential Care*, 14–15.

78 The concept of a "mixed economy" within the welfare state is outlined by Lewis, "Welfare State or Mixed Economy of Welfare?"

79 These administrative and political details are drawn from the following sources: BCA, GR 496, Box 49, File 8, P. Walker to P. Ward, 11 May 1942; Box 50, File 1, M.F. Hunter to G. Weir, 23 May 1940; McFarland, "The Care of the Chronically Ill," 24–5.

80 McFarland, "The Care of the Chronically Ill," 73–4. This was the same year that the Provincial Hospital Insurance Act was passed, creating the British Columbia Hospital Insurance Service and a premium payment plan to provide hospital care benefits for acute illness to provincial residents.

81 VCA-CR, Box 29, File 3, "Report, Health and Social Welfare Committee," 27 November 1944; BCA, GR 496, Box 18, File 15, G. Pearson to F. Winslaw, 1 December 1944.

82 BCA, GR 678, Box 10, File 25, E. Pringle, "The Need for Chronic Diseases Hospitals," 1953; GR 679, Box 3, File 8, Memo by D. Cox, 27 July 1956.

83 BCA, GR 678, Box 1, File 7, D. Cox to E. Martin, 17 February 1956.

84 Ibid., File 6, L. Detwiller to D. Cox, 3 February 1958.

85 Ibid., File 7, Press statement announcing the chronic care program, 16 March 1956.

86 Ibid., File 6, L. Detwiller to D. Cox, 3 February 1958.

87 Elizabeth B. Hurlock, "As We Live: Public Minded Citizens Urged to Investigate Nursing Homes," *Victoria Times*, 1953.
88 VCA-CR, Box 23, Files 4–5, "Reports of the Home Committee," 15 February 1936 and 1 April 1936; Box 27, File 3, "Report of the Home Committee," 4 February 1942; Box 28, File 1, "Report of the Home Committee," 22 April 1943.
89 Achenbaum, *Shades of Grey*, 39–40.
90 Patients at the Saanich Health Centre who received old age pensions were also required to turn their pension cheques over to the municipality. SMA, Clerk's Department, Box 87, File 3, J. Tribe to W. Greene, 8 August 1946. This was also the case in other areas of Canada. See Snell, "Maintenance Agreements for the Elderly," 197–216. Snell's work is excellent for illustrating how old age pensions were implemented within the older system of maintenance agreements for the aged.
91 VCA-CR, Box 24, File 3, "Report of the Home Committee," 1937; Box 27, File 3, "Home Committee Report," 4 February 1942.
92 BCA, GR 496, Box 49, File 5, "Annual Report of the Welfare Institutions Board for the Calendar Year 1946."
93 BCA, GR 678, Box 1, File 7, J. Mainguy to D. Cox, 14 May 1956.
94 Ibid., "Report on Percentage of Welfare Patients in Private Hospitals as at midnight April 15, 1956," and J. Mainguy to D. Cox, 14 May 1956. I also used Province of British Columbia, *Report on Hospital Statistics*, 1956.
95 BCA, GR 496, Box 49, File 5, Welfare Institutions Board Minutes, 22 September 1944.
96 BCA, GR 679, Box 3, File 38, D. Cox to E. Martin, 17 June 1955.
97 BCA, GR 678, Box 5, File 12, J. Mainguy to D. Cox, 30 October 1962. The government kept a close watch on private hospital ownership, limiting ownership to one establishment of fifty beds until 1960. At that point the policy was changed, allowing owners to have an interest in two institutions of seventy-five beds.
98 Ibid., Box 1, File 6, D. Cox to E. Martin, 26 November 1956.
99 Ibid., Box 10, File 25, F. Switzer to W.A.C. Bennett, 15 February 1955.
100 Ibid., G. Pelton to E. Martin, 14 February 1955.
101 This figure compares to a national average of 7.6 per cent of the population over the age of sixty-five in 1961. In B.C. this segment of the population had risen from 5.5 per cent in 1931. See Ward, "Population Growth in Western Canada," table 5, 171.
102 BCA, GR 678, Box 1, File 16. E. Martin to J.W. Duncan, 21 January 1964.
103 BCA, GR 679, Box 2, File 23, E. Martin to J. LaMarsh, 8 October 1964. Cox had alerted Martin to this possible loophole six months earlier. BCA, GR 678, Box 20, File 21, D. Cox to E. Martin, 24 March 1964.

CONCLUSION

1 Thomson, "The Decline of Social Welfare."
2 Thomson, "The Welfare of the Elderly in the Past."
3 For example, Thomson, "Welfare and the Historians"; Guillemard, "Introduction" to *Old Age and the Welfare State*, 3–15; Gratton, "The New History of the Aged: A Critique"; Myles, *Old Age in the Welfare State*.
4 Starr, *The Social Transformation*, 145.
5 This kind of intellectual configuration is used in the work of Adams, *Architecture in the Family Way*.

Bibliography

ARCHIVAL SOURCES

BRITISH COLUMBIA ARCHIVES (BCA)
Add. MSS. 2818, Local Council of Women, Victoria
GR 131, British Columbia, Provincial Home (Kamloops), 1895–1975
GR 150, British Columbia, Provincial Secretary, Records Concerning Indigents, 1910–1925
GR 277, British Columbia, Department of Health Services and Hospital Insurance, Hospital Insurance Division
GR 281, British Columbia, Department of Health and Welfare, Hospital Insurance Service, Originals, 1913–1957
GR 289, British Columbia, Provincial Secretary, Indigent Funds, Originals, 1914–1933
GR 496, British Columbia, Provincial Secretary, Originals, 1929–1947
GR 678, British Columbia, Department of Health, Deputy Minister of Medical and Hospital Programmes, Originals, 1946–1976
GR 679, British Columbia, Department of Health Services & Hospital Insurance, Hospital Insurance Service, Originals, 1948–1971
GR 738, British Columbia, Report and Evidence concerning the Commission of Inquiry into the Provincial Home, Kamloops, 1903–1904
GR 907, British Columbia, Report and Evidence concerning the Home of the Friendless (1937)
GR 911, British Columbia, Commission of Welfare Institutions and Nursing Homes (1938)

GR 1249, British Columbia, Old Age Pensions Department, Originals, 1927–1949

GR 1582, B.C. Register of Companies

GR 2577, British Columbia, Hospital Programs, Originals, 1949–1976

GR 2720, British Columbia, Department of Health and Welfare, Originals, 1941–1958

BRITISH COLUMBIA LEGISLATIVE LIBRARY (BCLL)

Amyot, G. "Hospital Control: An Address Given at the Staff Conference of the Health and Welfare Services of the Department of the Provincial Secretary on January 5, 1937."

Harvey, Isobel. "The Generalized Social Worker in Public Welfare – with Particular Reference to the Welfare Field Service of British Columbia." 1937

– "Study of Chronic Diseases in British Columbia." 1945

DIOCESE OF BRITISH COLUMBIA ARCHIVES

GORGE ROAD HOSPITAL FILES

J.L. Gayton, "Gorge Road Hospital History."

NATIONAL ARCHIVES OF CANADA (NA)

OAK BAY MUNICIPALITY (OB-DHM)

Clerk's Office, David Havard, "Memoir."

ROSE MANOR COLLECTION (RMC)

Rose Manor Minute Books

T. D. Whittier, "History of Aged and Infirm Women's Home from March 14, 1893 to October 1, 1952."

James Morton, "To My Neighbours of the Aged Women's Home" (1942)

SAANICH MUNICIPAL ARCHIVES (SMA)

Clerk's Department

Vertical Subject Files

SIMMONS COLLEGE ARCHIVES, BOSTON, MASS.

Simmons College Catalogues

SISTERS OF SAINT ANN ARCHIVES (SSAA)

Mount Saint Mary's Chronicles

Mount Saint Mary's Collection

Mount Saint Mary's Correspondence

UNIVERSITY OF TORONTO ARCHIVES (UTA)
B72–0022, Papers of Harry Morris Cassidy

VICTORIA CITY ARCHIVES (VCA)
City By-laws
City Reports
Clerk's Department, Series Man-4, Committee Reports, 1885–1956 (VCA-CR)
Fire Insurance Maps

VANCOUVER CITY ARCHIVES (VANCA)
Social Service Department fonds, Series 452, 106-FI Old People's Home
Records, 1907–1971

OTHER SOURCES

Abbott, Andrew. *The System of Professionals: An Essay on the Division of Expert Labor.* Chicago: University of Chicago Press 1988.
Achenbaum, W. Andrew. *Old Age in the New Land: The American Experience Since 1790.* Baltimore: Johns Hopkins University Press 1978.
– "Historical Gerontology Comes of Age." *International Journal of Aging and Human Development* 18, no. 4 (1983–84): 231–57.
– *Shades of Grey: Old Age, American Values and Federal Policies Since 1920.* Boston: Little and Brown 1983.
– *Crossing Frontiers: Gerontology Emerges as a Science.* Cambridge: Cambridge University Press 1995.
Adams, Annmarie. *Architecture in the Family Way: Doctors, Houses, and Women, 1870–1900.* Montreal and Kingston: McGill-Queen's University Press 1996.
Anderson, Michael. "The Impact on the Family Relationships of the Elderly of Changes Since Victorian Times in Government Income-Maintenance Provision." In *Family, Bureaucracy and the Elderly,* ed. Ethel Shanas. Durham, North Carolina: Duke University Press 1977.
Anderson, Robin John. "Sharks and Red Herrings: Vancouver's Male Employment Agencies, 1898–1915." *BC Studies* 98 (summer 1993): 43–84.
Armstrong, David. *Political Anatomy of the Body: Medical Knowledge in Britain in the Twentieth Century.* Cambridge: Cambridge University Press 1983.
Atwood, Margaret. *morning in the burned house: new poems.* Toronto: McClelland & Stewart 1995.
Baldwin, Norma, John Harris, and Des Kelly. "Institutionalisation: Why Blame the Institution?" *Ageing and Society* 13, no. 2 (1993): 69–81.
Barker, Dr Lewellys. "On the Care of the Aged." *Canadian Hospital* 18, no. 4 (April 1941): 31, 38.

Barman, Jean. *The West Beyond the West: A History of British Columbia.* Toronto: University of Toronto Press 1991.

Berton, Pierre. "25 Pensioners Happy at Mother Fowler's." *Vancouver Sun.* 24 October 1946, 13.

Bishop, Hazeldine. "Edmonton's Friendship Club." *Canadian Welfare* 25, no. 6 (December 1949): 41–2.

Blanchard, Paula. *The Life of Emily Carr.* Vancouver: Douglas and McIntyre 1987.

Boas, Ernest. *The Unseen Plague, Chronic Disease.* New York: J.J. Augustin 1940.

Bradbury, Bettina. *Working Families: Age, Gender and Daily Survival in Industrializing Montreal.* Toronto: McClelland & Stewart 1993.

Brown, E. Richard. *Rockefeller Medicine Men: Medicine and Capitalism in America.* Berkeley: University of California Press 1979.

Bryden, Kenneth. *Old Age Pensions and Policy-Making in Canada.* Montreal: McGill-Queen's University Press 1974.

Byron, David Bentley, John David Shillington, Utho Charles Stedidle, and Raymond John Thomlison. "The Social Welfare Philosophy of the Social Credit Party of British Columbia." Master's of Social Work thesis, University of British Columbia 1965.

Calder, James. "A Prescription for Longevity." *Alberta Medical Bulletin* 13, no. 4 (October 1948): 3–4.

Calm, John, ed. *Alex Lord's British Columbia: Recollections of a Rural School Inspector, 1915–1936.* Vancouver: University of British Columbia Press 1991.

Canadian Who's Who. Vol. 2. Ed. Charles Roberts. Toronto: Murray Publishing 1936.

Canadian Who's Who. Vol. 4. Toronto: Trans Canada Press 1948.

Cassidy, H.M. *Unemployment and Relief in Ontario, 1929–1932.* Toronto: J.M. Dent and Sons 1932.

– "British Columbia Provincial Workers Meet." *Child and Family Welfare* 12, no. 6 (March 1937): 48–50.

– "Personnel Changes in British Columbia." *Canadian Welfare Summary* 14, no. 4 (November 1938): 43–5.

– *Public Health and Welfare Reorganization: The Post-War Problem in the Canadian Provinces.* Toronto: Ryerson Press 1945.

Censuses of the Dominion of Canada, 1901–1961.

Christie, Agatha. *They Do It With Mirrors.* Glasgow: Fontana-Collins 1952.

Chudacoff, Howard P. and Tamara Hareven. "From the Empty Nest to Family Dissolution: Life Course Transitions into Old Age." *Journal of Family History* 4, no. 1 (spring 1979): 69–83.

Clough, Roger. *Old Age Homes.* London: George Allen 1981.

Coates, Colin M. "Death in British Columbia, 1850–1950." Master's thesis, University of British Columbia 1984.

Cohen, Anthony P. *The Symbolic Construction of Community.* London: Tavistock Press 1985.

Cohen, Marjorie Griffin. "The Decline of Women in Canadian Dairying." *Histoire sociale/Social History* 17, no. 34 (November 1984): 307–34.

Cole, Thomas R. *The Journey of Life: A Cultural History of Aging in America.* Cambridge: Cambridge University Press 1991.

– "The Spectre of Old Age: History, Politics, and Culture in an Aging America." In *Growing Old in America*, eds. Beth B. Hess and Elizabeth W. Markson. New Brunswick, New Jersey: Transaction Publications 1991.

Con, Harry, Ronald J. Con, Graham Johnson, Edgar Wickberg, and William E. Willmott. *From China to Canada: A History of the Chinese Communities in Canada.* Toronto: McClelland & Stewart 1982.

Conrad, Margaret. "Sundays Always Make Me Think of Home: Time and Place in Canadian Women's History." In *Not Just Pin Money: Selected Essays on the History of Women's Work in British Columbia*, eds. B. Latham and R. Pazdro. Victoria: Camosun College Press 1984.

Cook, Sharon Anne. "'A Quiet Place ... to Die': Ottawa's First Protestant Old Age Homes for Women and Men." *Ontario History* 81, no. 1 (March 1989): 25–40.

Corley-Smith, Peter. *White Bears and Other Curiosities ... The First 100 Years of the Royal British Columbia Museum.* Victoria: Royal British Columbia Museum 1989.

Creighton, J.H. "Birthdays Don't Count." *Canadian Welfare* 24, no. 8 (March 1949): 37–40.

Crowther, Anne. *The Workhouse System, 1834–1929: The History of an English Social Institution.* London: Batsford Academic and Educational Ltd 1981.

– *British Social Policy, 1914–1939.* Basingstoke: Macmillan Education Ltd 1988.

Daily Province (Vancouver)

Danysk, Cecilia. *Hired Hands: Labour and the Development of Prairie Agriculture.* Toronto: McClelland & Stewart 1995.

– "A Bachelor's Paradise." In *Making Western Canada: Essays on European Colonization and Settlement*, eds. Catherine Cavanaugh and Jeremy Mouat. Toronto: Garamond Press 1996.

Davies, Megan J. "Old Age in British Columbia: The Case of the 'Lonesome Prospector.'" *BC Studies* no. 118 (summer 1998): 41–66.

– "Mapping 'Region' in Canadian Medical History: The Case of British Columbia." *Canadian Bulletin of Medical History* 17 (2002): 73–92.

– "Competent Professionals and Modern Methods: State Medicine in British Columbia during the 1930s." *Bulletin of the History of Medicine* 76, no. 1 (spring 2002): 56–83.

Demos, John. "Aging in Pre-Modern Society: The Case of Early New England." In *Aging, Death and the Completion of Being*, ed. D. Van Tassel. Philadelphia: University of Pennsylvania Press 1979.

Dennis, Richard and Stephen Daniels. "Community and the Social Geography of Victorian Cities." In *Time, Family and Community: Perspectives on Family and Community History*, ed. Michael Drake. Milton Keynes: Open University Press 1994.

Dillon, Lisa. "Your Place or Mine? Household Arrangements of Widows and Widowers in Nineteenth-Century Ottawa: A Study of Three Wards." Paper presented at the Canadian Historical Conference, Charlottetown, June 1992.

Du Moulin, Anne. "Gordon House Serves Its Senior Citizens." *Canadian Welfare* 25, no. 6 (December 1949): 26–30.

Ehrenreich, John H. *The Altruistic Imagination: A History of Social Work and Social Policy in the United States*. Ithaca: Cornell University Press 1985.

Elmore, Eugene. "Discharge Planning in Homes for the Aged: An Analytical Survey of a Group of Patients Hospitalized for Mental Illness in the Homes for the Aged, Port Coquitlam, B.C." Master's of Social Work thesis, University of British Columbia 1959.

Farquhar, H.S. "Services for the Aged." *Proceedings of the 10th Biennial Meeting of the Canadian Conference on Social Work* (1946): 109–12.

Finlayson, Geoffrey. *Citizen, State and Social Welfare in Britain, 1830–1990*. Oxford: Clarendon Press 1994.

Fischer, David Hackett. *Growing Old in America*. Oxford: Oxford University Press 1978.

Fisher, Robin. *Duff Pattullo of British Columbia*. Toronto: University of Toronto Press 1991.

Forbes, William, Jennifer A. Jackson, and Arthur S. Kraus. *Institutionalization of the Elderly in Canada*. Toronto: Butterworths 1987.

Forestell, Nancy. "Bachelors, Boarding-Houses and Blind Pigs." In *A Nation of Immigrants: Women, Workers and Communities in Canadian History, 1840s-1960s*, eds. Paula Draper, Franca Iacovetta, and Robert Ventresca. Toronto: University of Toronto Press 1998.

Forty, Adrian. "The Modern Hospital in England and France: The Social and Medical Uses of Architecture." In *Buildings and Society: Essays on the Social Development of the Built Environment*, ed. Anthony D. King. London: Routledge and Kegan Paul 1980.

Freeden, Michael. *The New Liberalism: An Ideology of Social Reform*. Oxford: Clarendon Press 1978.

Goffman, Erving. *Asylums: Essays on the Social Situation of Mental Patients and Other Inmates*. New York: Anchor Books 1961.

Gordon, Chris. "Familial Support for the Elderly in the Past: The Case of London's Working Class in the Early 1930s." *Ageing and Society* 8, no. 4 (1988): 287–320.

Gordon, Linda. *Heroes of Their Own Lives: The Politics and History of Family Violence.* London: Penguin Books 1988.

– "The New Feminist Scholarship on the Welfare State." In *Women, the State, and Welfare,* ed. Linda Gordon. Madison, Wisconsin: University of Wisconsin Press, 1990.

Gould, Ida. *History of the Aged and Infirm Women's Home, Victoria, British Columbia, 1897–1928.* Victoria: King's Printer 1928.

Graebner, William. *A History of Retirement: The Meaning and Function of An American Institution, 1885–1978.* New Haven: Yale University Press 1980.

– "The Golden Age Clubs." *Social Service Review* 57, no. 3 (September 1983): 416–28.

Grainger, M. Allerdale. *Woodsmen of the West.* Toronto: McClelland & Stewart 1996.

Gratton, Brian. "Social Workers and Old Age Pensions." *Social Service Review* 57, no. 3 (September 1983): 403–15.

– "The New History of the Aged: A Critique." In *Old Age in a Bureaucratic Society: The Elderly, the Experts, and the State in American History,* eds. David Van Tassel and Peter N. Stearns. New York: Greenwood Press 1986.

Gresko, Jacqueline. "Salomée Valois." In *Dictionary of Canadian Biography* Vol. 13 (1901–1910): 1048–9.

Gubrium, Jaber F. *Living and Dying at Murray Manor.* New York: St Martin's Press 1975.

Guest, Dennis. "Taylor Manor – A Survey of the Facilities of Vancouver's Home for the Aged." Master's of Social Work thesis, University of British Columbia 1952.

– *The Emergence of Social Security in Canada.* Vancouver: University of British Columbia Press 1980.

Guildford, Janet. "Closing the Mansions of Woe: The End of the Poor Law in Nova Scotia, 1944–1965." Paper presented at the Canadian Historical Conference, St John's, June 1997.

Guillemard, Anne-Marie, ed. *Old Age and the Welfare State.* London: SAGE Publications 1983.

Haber, Carole. *Beyond Sixty-Five: The Dilemma of Old Age in America's Past.* Cambridge: Cambridge University Press 1983.

Hareven, Tamara. "The Last Stage: Historical Adulthood and Old Age." *Daedalus* 105 (1976): 13–27.

– "Life-Course Transitions and Kin Assistance in Old Age: A Cohort Comparison." In *Old Age in a Bureaucratic Society: The Elderly, the Experts, and the State in American History,* eds. David Van Tassel and Peter N. Stearns. New York: Greenwood Press 1986.

Harney, Robert F. "Men Without Women: Italian Migrants in Canada, 1885–1930." In *A Nation of Immigrants: Women, Workers and Communities in*

Canadian History, 1840s-1960s, eds. Paula Draper, Franca Iacovetta, and Robert Ventresca. Toronto: University of Toronto Press 1998.

Harris, Cole. "Industry and the Good Life around Idaho Peak." In *The Resettlement of British Columbia: Essays on Colonialism and Geographical Change.* Vancouver: UBC Press 1997.

Hill, Ruth. "Old People Have a Future." *Proceedings: Canadian Conference on Social Work* (1950): 147–52.

Himmelfarb, Gertrude. *The Idea of Poverty: England in the Early Industrial Age.* London: Faber and Faber 1984.

Hinde, John R. "Stout Ladies and Amazons: Women in the British Columbia Coal-Mining Community of Ladysmith, 1912–1914." *BC Studies* no. 114 (summer 1997): 33–58.

Holland, Laura. "Our Senior Citizens." *Canadian Welfare* 20, no. 6 (December 1944): 26–7.

Hunt, E.M. "Paupers and Pensioners: Past and Present." *Ageing and Society* 9, no. 4 (1990): 407–30.

Hutchison, Bruce. *The Unknown Country: Canada and Her People.* Toronto: Longmans, Green and Co. 1943.

Irving, Allan. "The Development of a Provincial Welfare State: British Columbia, 1900–1939." In *The 'Benevolent' State: The Growth of Welfare in Canada*, eds. Allan Moscovitch and Jim Albert. Toronto: Garamond Press 1987.

– "Canadian Fabians: The Work and Thought of Harry Cassidy and Leonard Marsh, 1930–1945." *CJSWE/rcess* 7, no. 1 (1981): 7–28.

Janeway, Elizabeth. *Powers of the Weak.* New York: Morrow Quill Paperbacks 1981.

Jerrome, Dorthy. "Me Darby, You Joan!" In *Dependency and Interdependency in Old Age: Theoretical Perspectives and Policy Alternatives*, eds. Chris Phillipson, Miriam Bernard, and Patricia Strang. London: Croom Helm 1986.

Johnson, Wingate M. "Old Age: A Public Health Problem." *Canadian Journal of Public Health* 38, no. 10 (October 1947): 461–8.

Johnston, Hugh. "Native People, Settlers and Sojourners, 1871–1916." In *The Pacific Province: A History of British Columbia*, ed. Hugh M. Johnston. Vancouver: Douglas and McIntyre 1996.

Katz, Michael B. *Poverty and Policy in American History.* New York: Academic Press 1983.

– "Poorhouses and the Origins of the Public Old Age Home." *Milbank Memorial Fund Quarterly* 62, no. 1 (1984): 110–40.

Kayser-Jones, Jeanie Schmit. *Old, Alone, and Neglected: Care of the Aged in Scotland and the United States.* Berkeley: University of California Press 1981.

Kelm, Mary-Ellen. "'The Only Place Likely to Do Her Any Good': The Admission of Women to British Columbia's Provincial Hospital for the Insane." *BC Studies* no. 96 (winter 1992–93): 66–89.

King, Anthony D., ed. *Buildings and Society: Essays on the Social Development of the Built Environment.* London: Routledge and Kegan Paul 1980.

Knight, Rolf. *A Very Ordinary Life.* Vancouver: New Star Books 1974.

– *Along the No. 20 Line: Reminiscences of the Vancouver Waterfront.* Vancouver: New Star Books 1980.

Kosa, John. *Land of Choice.* Toronto: University of Toronto Press 1957.

Krasnick Warsh, Cheryl. *Moments of Unreason: The Practice of Canadian Psychiatry and the Homewood Retreat, 1883–1923.* Montreal: McGill-Queen's University Press 1989.

Kreiger, E. "An Introduction to Geriatrics." *University of Toronto Medical Journal* 24, no. 3 (December 1946): 67–9.

Kunzel, Regina G. *Fallen Women, Problem Girls: Unmarried Mothers and the Professionalization of Social Work, 1890–1945.* New Haven: Yale University Press 1993.

Lai, David Chueyan. "From Self-segregation to Integration: The Vicissitudes of Victoria's Chinese Hospital." *BC Studies* no. 80 (winter 1988–89): 52–68.

Lansdowne, Rosemary. "B.C. Field Service Grows Up: A One-Act Play." *Canadian Welfare* 24, no. 6 (December 1948): 20–6.

Laslett, Peter. "The Traditional English Family and the Aged in our Society." In *Aging, Death and the Completion of Being,* ed. D. Van Tassel. Philadelphia: University of Pennsylvania Press 1979.

Laurence, Margaret. *The Stone Angel.* Toronto: McClelland & Stewart 1968.

Leigh, Amy. "Public Welfare in British Columbia." *Proceedings of the Ninth Canadian Conference on Social Work* (1944): 133–5.

Letter to the Editor. *The Canadian Doctor* 15, no. 9 (September 1949): 4.

Lewis, Jane. "Welfare State or Mixed Economy of Welfare?" *History Today* 45, no. 2 (1995): 4–6.

Lewis, Jane and Barbara Meredith. "Daughters Caring for Mothers: the Experience of Caring and its Implications for Professional Helpers." *Ageing and Society* 8, no. 1 (1988): 1–21.

Leydier, Bernice. "Boarding Home Care for the Aged: A Study of the Social Welfare Aspects of Licensed Homes in Vancouver." Master's of Social Work thesis, University of British Columbia 1948.

Li, Peter S. *The Chinese in Canada.* Toronto: Oxford University Press 1988.

Lugrin, N. de Bertrand. *The Pioneer Women of Vancouver Island, 1843–1866.* Victoria: Women's Canadian Club of Victoria 1928.

McDonald, Robert A.J. *Making Vancouver: Class, Status and Social Boundaries, 1863–1913.* Vancouver: UBC Press 1996.

McFarland, William Donald. "The Care of the Chronically Ill: A Survey of the Existing Facilities and Needs Of Vancouver." Master's of Social Work thesis, University of British Columbia 1948.

McLaren, Arlene Tigar. "Family Life." In *Working Lives: Vancouver, 1886–1986,* eds. The Working Lives Collective. Vancouver: New Star Books 1985.

MacPherson, Dr J. Interview with Brenda Davies. Victoria, British Columbia. October 1990. Private collection of the author.

MacQuarrie, Bruce McKenzie. "The Care of An Ageing and Disabled Group in a Veterans Hospital: An Appraisal of the Domiciliary Care Programme Provided by the Department of Veterans' Affairs in Vancouver." Master's of Social Work thesis, University of British Columbia 1950.

Markus, Thomas A. *Buildings and Power: Freedom and Control in the Origin of Modern Building Types.* London: Routledge 1993.

Mathewson, Eleanor Weld. "Old Age Pensions in British Columbia: A Review of Trends in Eligibility." Master's in Social Work thesis, University of British Columbia 1949.

May, Elaine Tyler. *Homeward Bound: American Families in the Cold War Era.* New York: Basic Books 1988.

Means, Robin and Randall Smith. *The Development of Welfare Services for Elderly People.* London: Croom Helm 1985.

– *From Poor Law to Community Care: The Development of Welfare Services for Elderly People, 1939–1971.* Bristol: The Policy Press 1998.

Moffatt, Ken. *A Poetics of Social Work: Personal Agency and Social Transformation in Canada, 1920–1939.* Toronto: University of Toronto Press 2001.

Montigny, Edgar-André. *Foisted upon the Government?: State Responsibilities, Family Obligations, and the Care of the Dependent Aged in Late Nineteenth-Century Ontario.* Montreal: McGill-Queen's University Press 1997.

Morton, Suzanne. "Old Women and their Place in Nova Scotia, 1881–1931." Paper presented at the Third Radall Symposium on Atlantic Literature and Culture, Acadia University, Wolfville, Nova Scotia, September 1992.

– *Ideal Surroundings: Gender and Domestic Life in a Working Class Suburb in the 1920s.* Toronto: University of Toronto Press 1995.

Mouat, Jeremy. *Roaring Days: Rossland's Mines and the History of British Columbia.* Vancouver: UBC Press 1995.

Muncy, Robyn. *Creating a Female Dominion: American Reform, 1890–1935.* New York: Oxford University Press 1991.

Myles, John. "Comparative Public Policies for the Elderly: Frameworks and Resources for Analysis." In *Old Age and the Welfare State*, ed. Anne-Marie Guillemard. London: SAGE Publications 1983.

– *Old Age in the Welfare State: The Political Economy of Public Pensions.* Lawrence, Kansas: University of Kansas Press 1989.

Nash, Bernard E. and Ethel McClure. "Aging in Retrospect." In *Aging in Minnesota*, ed. Arnold M. Rose. Minneapolis: University of Minnesota Press 1963.

"New Developments in British Columbia's Health and Welfare Services." *Child and Family* 11, no. 1 (May 1935): 35–9.

"News Notes." *Canadian Nurse* 41, no. 1 (January 1945):69.

Novak, Mark. *Aging and Society: A Canadian Perspective.* Scarborough, Ontario: Nelson 1993.

- "Old Age Welfare." *Canadian Doctor* 11, no. 10 (October 1945): 40, 42–3.
Ormsby, Margaret. *British Columbia: A History.* Vancouver: Evergreen Press 1958.
Owram, Doug. *The Government Generation: Canadian Intellectuals and the State, 1900–1945.* Toronto: University of Toronto Press 1986.
Parker, R.A. *The Elderly and Residential Care: Australian Lessons for Britain.* Aldershot, Hants.: Gower Publishing Ltd 1987.
Parr, Joy. *The Gender of Breadwinners: Men, Women and Change in Two Industrial Towns, 1880–1950.* Toronto: University of Toronto Press 1990.
Paulson, Esther. "East Kootenay Health and Welfare Service, 1935–38." *B.C. Historical News* (fall 1997): 17–21.
Peace, Sheila, Leonie Kellaher, and Dianne Willcocks. *Re-evaluating Residential Care.* Buckingham, England: Open University Press 1997.
Perkin, Harold. *The Rise of Professional Society: England since 1880.* London: Routledge 1989.
Perry, Adele. "'Oh I'm Just Sick of the Faces of Men': Gender Imbalance, Race, Sexuality, and Sociability in Nineteenth-Century British Columbia." *BC Studies* 105–106 (spring/summer 1995): 27–44.
Phillips, Jock. *A Man's Country: The Image of the Pakeha Male – A History.* Auckland: Penguin Books 1987.
Phillipson, Chris. *Capitalism and the Construction of Old Age.* London: Macmillan Press 1982.
Pringle, Edith. "British Columbia Shows the Way." *Canadian Nurse* 37, no. 11 (November 1941): 749–51.
Province of British Columbia. Department of the Provincial Secretary. *Hospital Service and Costs, 1934.* Victoria: King's Printer 1935.
- Provincial Board of Health. *Public Health Nursing, British Columbia, Canada.* Victoria: King's Printer 1925.
- Department of the Provincial Secretary. *Hospital Statistics and Administration of the "Hospital Act."* Victoria: King's Printer, various dates.
- Department of Health and Welfare. *Report on Hospital Statistics.* Various dates.
"Public Welfare in British Columbia." *Canadian Welfare* 22, no. 2 (June 1946): 2–6.
Quadagno, Jill. *The Transformation of Old Age Security: Class and Politics in the American Welfare State.* Chicago: University of Chicago Press 1988.
Quadagno, Jill and Madonna Harrington-Meyer. "Organized Labor, State Structures, and Social Policy Development: A Case Study of Old Age Assistance in Ohio, 1916–1940." *Social Problems* 36, no. 2 (April 1989): 181–96.
Reaume, Geoffrey. "Portraits of People with Mental Disorders in English Canadian History." *Canadian Bulletin of Medical History* 17, nos 1–2 (2000): 93–125.
Roberts, David. *Paternalism in Early Victorian England.* London: Croom Helm 1979.

Robin, Jean. "Family Care of the Elderly in a Nineteenth-Century Devonshire Parish." *Ageing and Society* 4, no. 4 (1984): 505–16.

Rogers, Stan. "First Christmas Away from Home." *Between the Breaks – Live!* Sound recording. Fogarty's Cove Music 1979.

Rosenberg, Charles. "Inward Vision and Outward Glance: The Shaping of the American Hospital." *Bulletin of the History of Medicine* 53, no. 3 (fall 1979): 346–91.

Rothman, David J. *The Discovery of the Asylum: Social Order and Disorder in the New Republic.* Boston: Little, Brown and Company 1971.

Rowe, Edith, Jane LeWare, and Jessie Wilson. "The Care of the Chronically Ill." *Canadian Nurse* 43, no. 8 (August 1947): 596–8.

Roy, Patricia. "Vancouver: 'The Mecca of the Unemployed,' 1907–1929." In *Town and Country: Aspects of Western Canadian Urban Development*, ed. Alan Artibise. Regina: University of Regina, 1981.

Rudy, Norma. *For Such a Time as This: L. Earl Ludlow and a History of Homes for the Aged in Ontario, 1837–1961.* Toronto: Ontario Association of Homes for the Aged 1987.

Sager, Eric and Peter Baskerville. *Unwilling Idlers: The Urban Unemployed and Their Families in Late-Victorian Canada.* Toronto: University of Toronto Press 1998.

Samson, Emily D. *Old Age in the New World.* London: The Pilot Press 1944.

Seager, Allan. "The Resource Economy, 1871–1921." In *The Pacific Province: A History of British Columbia*, ed. Hugh Johnson. Vancouver: Douglas and McIntyre 1996.

Sessional Papers, British Columbia. (SP)

Simmons, Beth and Vic. Interview with Brenda Davies. Victoria, British Columbia. October 1990. Private collection of the author.

Skocpol, Theda. *Protecting Soldiers and Mothers: The Political Origins of Social Policy in the United States.* Cambridge: The Belknap Press of Harvard University Press 1992.

Smith, Daniel Scott. "Life Course, Norms, and the Family System of Older Americans in 1900." *Journal of Family History* 4, no. 3 (fall 1978): 285–90.

– "Accounting for Change in the Families of the Elderly in the United States, 1900-Present." *Old Age in a Bureaucratic Society: The Elderly, the Experts, and the State in American History*, eds. David Van Tassel and Peter N. Stearns. New York: Greenwood Press 1986.

Smith, Daniel Scott, Michael Dahlin, and Mark Friedberger. "The Family Structure of the Older Black Population in the American South in 1880 and 1900." *Sociology and Social Research* 63, no. 3 (1977): 544–65.

Smith, James E. "Widowhood and Ageing in Traditional English Society." *Ageing and Society* 4, no. 4 (1984): 429–49.

Smith, Richard M. "The Structured Dependence of the Elderly as a Recent Development: Some Sceptical Historical Thoughts." *Ageing and Society* 4, no. 4 (1984): 409–27.

Snell, James. "Maintenance Agreements for the Elderly: Canada, 1900–1951." *Journal of the Canadian Historical Association / Revue de la Société historique du Canada* (1992): 197–216.

– "The First Grey Lobby: The Old Age Pensioners' Organization of British Columbia, 1932–1951." BC *Studies* no. 102 (summer 1994): 3–29.

– *The Citizen's Wage: The State and the Elderly in Canada, 1900–1951*. Toronto: University of Toronto Press 1996.

Social Planning and Research Council of B.C. and United Way Research Services. *The Learnings From the New Horizons, Partners in Aging Projects: Final Report*. Vancouver: SPARC April 1997.

Special Committee of Montreal Social Workers (Mrs M.A. Lanthier, Chairman). *The Case of the Chronically Ill in Montreal*. Metropolitan Life Insurance Company 1941.

Starr, Paul. *The Social Transformation of American Medicine*. New York: Basic Books 1982.

Stevens, Rosemary. *In Sickness and in Wealth: American Hospitals in the Twentieth Century*. New York: Basic Books 1989.

Stewart, Stormi. "The Elderly Poor in Rural Ontario: Inmates of the Wellington County House of Industry, 1877–1907." *Journal of the Canadian Historical Association / Revue de la Société historique du Canada*. (1992): 217–33.

Stone, Lawrence. *The Past and Present Revisited*. London: Routledge and Kegan Paul 1987.

Strong-Boag, Veronica. *The New Day Recalled: Lives of Girls and Women in English Canada, 1919–1939*. Toronto: Copp Clark Pitman 1988.

– "Home Dreams: Women and the Suburban Experiment in Canada, 1945–60." *Canadian Historical Review* 72, no. 4 (December 1991): 471–504.

Strong-Boag, Veronica and Kathryn McPherson. "The Confinement of Women: Childbirth and Hospitalization in Vancouver, 1919–1939." BC *Studies* nos 69–70 (spring/summer 1986): 142–74.

Struthers, James. "Lord Give Us Men: Women and Social Work in English Canada, 1918 to 1953." *Historical Papers* (1983): 96–112.

– "A Profession in Crisis: Charlotte Whitton and Canadian Social Work in the 1930s." In *The 'Benevolent' State: The Growth of Welfare in Canada*, eds. Allan Moscovitch and Jim Albert. Toronto: Garamond Press 1987.

– "Regulating the Elderly: Old Age Pensions and the Formation of a Pension Bureaucracy in Ontario, 1929–1945." *Journal of the Canadian Historical Association / Revue de la Société historique du Canada* (1992): 235–55.

– *The Limits of Affluence: Welfare in Ontario, 1920–1970*. Toronto: University of Toronto Press 1994.

Sundstrom, Gerdt. "Family and State: Recent Trends in the Care of the Aged in Sweden." *Ageing and Society* 6 (1986): 169–96.

Synge, Jane. "Work and Family Support Patterns of the Aged in the Early Twentieth Century." In *Aging in Canada: Social Perspectives*, ed. Victor W. Marshall. Don Mills, Ontario: Fitzhenry and Whiteside 1980.

Talker, Elizabeth. "Services for Married Couples on Assistance and Pension: A Type Study of a Selected Group of Cases in Vancouver." Master's of Social Work thesis, University of British Columbia 1956.

Tamke, Susan S. "Human Values and Aging: The Perspective of the Victorian Nursery." In *Aging and the Elderly: Humanistic Perspectives in Gerontology*, eds. S. Spicker, K.Woodward, and D. Van Tassel. New Jersey: Humanistic Press 1978.

Taylor, John. "The Urban West, Public Welfare, and a Theory of Urban Development." In *Cities in the West*, eds. A.R. McCormack and I. Macpherson. Ottawa: National Museum of Man 1975.

Tennant, M. "Elderly Indigents and Old Men's Homes, 1880–1920." *New Zealand Journal of History* 17 (1983): 3–20.

Thane, Pat. "Geriatrics." In *Companion Encylcopedia of the History of Medicine*, vol. 2, eds. W.F. Bynum and Roy Porter. London and New York: Routledge, 1997.

– *Old Age in English History: Past Experiences, Present Issues*. Oxford: Oxford University Press 2000.

Thompson, John and Grace Goldin. *The Hospital: A Social and Architectural History*. Yale: Yale University Press 1973.

Thomson, David. "Workhouse to Nursing Home: Residential Care of Elderly people in England since 1840." *Ageing and Society* 3, no. 2 (1983): 43–69.

– "The Decline of Social Welfare: Falling State Support for the Elderly since Early Victorian Times." *Ageing and Society* 4, no. 4 (1984): 451–82.

– "Welfare and the Historians." In *The World We Have Gained: Histories of Population and Social Structure*, eds. Lloyd Bondfield, Richard M. Smith, and Keith Wrightson. Oxford: Basil Blackwell, 1986.

– "The Welfare of the Elderly in the Past: A Family or Community Responsibility?" In *Life, Death and the Elderly: Historical Perspectives*, eds. Margaret Pelling and Richard M. Smith. London: Routledge 1991.

Tobin, Sheldon S. and Morton A. Lieberman. *Last Home for the Aged: Critical Implications of Institutionalization*. San Francisco: Jossey-Bass 1976.

Townsend, Peter. *The Family Life of Old People: An Inquiry in East London*. London: Routledge and Kegan Paul 1957.

– *The Last Refuge: A Survey of Residential Institutions for the Aged in England and Wales*. London: Routledge and Kegan Paul 1964.

– "The Structured Dependency of the Elderly: A Creation of Social Policy in the Twentieth Century." *Ageing and Society* 1, no. 1 (1981): 6–28.

Tysoe, J.F. "An Integrated Community Programme for Rehabilitation: Rehabilitation of the Aged." *Proceedings: Canadian Conference on Social Work* (1950): 144–7.

– "University of British Columbia Plans Special Training." *Canadian Welfare* 20, no. 1 (April 1944): 29.

Vancouver News Herald

Vancouver Sun

Victoria and Vancouver Island Directory (1952). Vancouver: B.C. Directories Ltd 1952.

Wade, Jill. *Houses for All: The Struggle for Social Housing in Vancouver, 1919–50*. Vancouver: UBC Press 1994.

Wagner, Margaret. "New Patterns for Old Age." *Proceedings of the 11th Biennial Meeting of the Canadian Conference on Social Work* (1948): 63–71.

Walker, T.W. "Better Provision Needed for the Chronically Ill." *Canadian Hospital* 23, no. 1 (January 1946): 34.

Ward, Percy. "How Much Hospitalization is Really Necessary for the Chronically Ill?" *Canadian Hospital* 23, no. 1 (January 1946): 35.

Ward, W. Peter. "Population Growth in Western Canada, 1901–1971." In *The Developing West: Essays on Canadian History in Honor of Lewis H. Thomas*, ed. John E. Foster. Edmonton: University of Alberta Press 1983.

Ware, Susan. *Beyond Suffrage: Women in the New Deal*. Cambridge: Harvard University Press 1981.

Webster, Charles. "The Elderly and the Early National Health Service." In *Life, Death, and the Elderly: Historical Perspectives*, eds. Margaret Pelling and Richard M. Smith. London: Routledge 1991.

Weiler, N. Sue. "Family Security or Social Security? The Family and the Elderly in New York State during the 1920s." *Journal of Family History* 11, no. 1 (1986): 76–95.

Weiss, Gillian. "An Essential Year for the Child: The Kindergarden in British Columbia." In *Schooling and Society in Twentieth Century British Columbia*, eds. J. Donald Wilson and David C. Jones. Calgary: Detselig Enterprises Limited 1980.

– "Where old people are understood." *Canadian Welfare* 24, no. 5 (15 October 1948): 29.

Wynn, Graeme. "The Rise of Vancouver." In *Vancouver and Its Region*, eds. Graeme Wynn and Timothy Oke. Vancouver: UBC Press 1992.

Young, George, M.D. "Growing Old Gracefully." *Canadian Nurse* 41, no. 1 (January 1945): 25–8.

Index

Old People's Home (Taylor Manor,
Vancouver), 12, 56, 60–2, 72, 100,
103, 115, 170; administration, 61;
institutional finances and patient
money, 115; and the local community,
138, 140–2, 171–2; location of, 61;
patient discontent and resistance,
127–9; patient illness and death,
130–2; patient labour, 120–4; physical description, 61; population, 61,
110; recreation, 141; redecoration,
61, 96–7; staff kindness to residents,
132–5; use of alcohol, 129, 140–1
old women: and children, 36–40, 172;
and community support, 34–5; and
daughters, 38–40, 135–8; and family, 16, 135–6, 172; lack of institutional facilities for women, 66;
marriage, 35–6; operating boarding
houses, 32; and poverty, 33–4; and
property, 32; single, 30–5; widowhood, 33; and work, 32–3
outdoor relief. See Indigent Fund

Page, Edna, 155
paternalism: in old age homes, 93; in
Poor Law treatment of the aged, 6,
45–7; in welfare state treatment of
the aged, 6, 50
Pattullo, T.D., 145, 147, 158, 160
Paulcer, Leo, 19
Perkin, Harold, 8
Phillipson, Chris, 9, 52
physiotherapy, 87, 92, 98–9, 101
Pioneer Home (Prince Rupert), 76, 96
pioneers, the concept of "worthy
pioneers," 6, 41, 171
Prince Rupert, 76
Pringle, Edith, 11, 154–5, 168
poor law: hatred of, 13; history of poor
law provision for the aged in central
and eastern Canada, 6–7; history
of the English Poor Law, 4–6, 171;
legacy of the English Poor Law in
B.C.'s old age homes, 4, 6–7, 75, 57,
87, 92, 114–30, 142–3; poor law
ethos in early B.C. state assistance,
45–7; poor law institutional provision in B.C., as compared to Ontario
and the Maritimes, 55; principle of
"less eligibility," 5, 115

professionalism in the old age home,
7–8, 54–85, 101–6
property: and old men alone, 26; and
old women alone, 32, and provincial
Indigent Fund, 47
Provincial Home for Aged Men (Kamloops), 11, 41–2, 58–60, 59, 73–4,
92, 95, 100, 110–12, 115, 116, 126–
7, 129, 170, 172; architecture and
design, 59–60; décor, 59–60; establishment of infirmary at Home, 60;
increasing numbers of infirm residents, 113; institutional finances and
patient money, 115; patient death,
131–2; patient labour, 120–3, 134;
patient population in Home, 59,
110–12; physical setting of Home,
59; routine, discipline and punishment, 117–19, 128–9; seasonal use
of the institution, 123–4; staff kindness to residents, 132–5
Provincial Home for Incurables (Provincial Infirmary at Marpole, Vancouver), 11, 62–3, 63, 77, 94–5, 102,
129, 172; administration and staff,
62, 106; architecture, 62; and institutional reforms, 89–90, 106; as key
site for professionalization, 89–94;
and local community, 139; nutrition,
93–4; occupational therapy, 92–4,
98–9, 106; overcrowding, 62, 113;
patient death, 131; patient discontent, 126; patient population, 62–3,
113; physical setting, 62; physiotherapy, 92–4, 98–9; and public opinion, 87; redecoration, 96–7; staff
kindness to residents, 132, 134–5;
women's auxiliary, 62–3, 92, 100,
141
Provincial Infirmary System (B.C.), 11,
72–5, 115, 162; Infirmary Advisory
Board, 89; institutional finances and
patient money, 115
provincial inspector of hospitals (B.C.),
82, 149
provincial police: as gatekeepers to institutions, 88; support for the elderly,
40, 42–3
Provincial Welfare Field Service, 89,
150–1; and the creation of geriatric
specialization, 151, 155; and gender,

provincial state bureaucracy, 146,
150–2, 155; as social workers, 88
Women's Auxiliaries in old age homes,
62–3, 92, 96–7, 100, 141
work: in old age for men, 27–30; in old
age for women, 32–3
workhouse: the institution in central
and eastern Canada, 7; not developing in B.C., 55
Workmen's Compensation Board, 50
Wynn, Graeme, 43

YMCA (Vancouver), 141